Bonnie C. Minsky, M.A., M.P.H., C.N.S., is an internationally recognized nutritionist who has been in private practice for almost 20 years. With a research background in teaching, school and family counseling, and public health education, she brings a unique, holistic perspective to her practice. Her first book, *Nutrition in a Nutshell* (Vital Health Publishing, 1999), was an informative and comprehensive approach to enhanced health through diet and supplementation. Ms. Minsky is a mother of three grown children and has three grandsons. Her extended family is a living example of the health benefits outlined in this book.

Dr. Lisa E. Holk, a Naturopathic physician, educator, and alternative medicine consultant, is currently on the faculty of Pacific College of Oriental Medicine and Chicago School of Massage Therapy. A member of the American Association of Naturopathic Physicians, Dr. Holk is currently licensed to practice in the State of Oregon. Patients, students, and colleagues alike are gratified by her thoughtful counsel on the achievement of optimal health through the modalities of alternative medicine. Dr. Holk applies her educational skills towards curriculum development, academic advisement, and consultative case management within the holistic model.

MORE VITAL HEALTH TITLES:

Trace Your Genes to Health (new 2nd ed.), Chris Reading, M.D., 336 pages, 1-890612-23-5, $15.95.

Smart Nutrients (new 2nd ed.), Abram Hoffer, M.D., Ph.D., Morton Walker, D.P.M., 224 pages, 1-890612-26-X, $14.95.

Stevia Sweet Recipes: Sugar-Free - Naturally! (2nd ed.), Jeffrey Goettemoeller, 200 pages, 1-890612-13-8, $13.95.

The Asthma Breakthrough: Breathe Freely – Naturally! Henry Osiecki, B.Sc., 192 pages, 1-890612-22-7, $13.95.

Nutrition in a Nutshell: Build Health and Slow Down the Aging Process, Bonnie Minsky, L.C.N., M.A., 196 pages, 1-890612-17-0, $14.95.

Wheatgrass: Superfood for a New Millenium, Li Smith, 164 pages, 1-890612-10-3, $10.95.

Energy For Life: How to Overcome Chronic Fatigue, George Redmon, Ph.D., N.D. approx. 240 pages, 1-890612-14-6, $15.95.

The Cancer Handbook: What's Really Working, edited by Lynne McTaggart, 192 pages, 1-890612-18-9, $12.95.

Taste Life! The Organic Choice, Ed. by David Richard and Dorie Byers, R.N., 208 pages, 1-890612-08-1, $12.95.

Healthy Living: A Holistic Guide to Cleansing, Revitalization and Nutrition, Susana Lombard, 112 pages, 1-890612-30-8, $12.95.

Stevia Rebaudiana: Nature's Sweet Secret, (3rd ed.) David Richard, 80 pages, 1-890612-15-4, $7.95. Includes growing info.

Healing Herb Rapid Reference, Brent Davis, D.C., 148 pages, 1-890612-21-9, $12.95.

Natural Beauty Basics: Making Your Own Cosmetics and Body Care Products, Dorie Byers, R.N., 208 pages, 1-890612-19-7, $14.95.

OUR CHILDREN'S HEALTH

America's Kids
in Nutritional Crisis
and What We Can Do
to Help Them

Bonnie C. Minsky
M.P.H., M.A., C.N.S., L.N.C.

WITH Lisa E. Holk
N.D., L.M.T.

VITAL HEALTH PUBLISHING
Ridgefield, CT

Cover design by David Richard
Interior design and production: Woodshed Productions

Our Children's Health: American's Kids in Nutritional Crisis and What We Can Do to Help Them

Copyright ©2002, Bonnie C. Minsky

Publisher's Cataloging-in-Publication
(Provided by Quality Books, Inc.)

Minsky, Bonnie C.
    Our children's health : American's kids in nutritional crisis and what we can do to help them / Bonnie C. Minsky, Lisa E. Holk. – 1st ed.
        p. cm.
    Includes bibliographical references
    ISBN: 1-890612-27-8

    1. Children—United States—Nutrition. I. Holk, Lisa E. II. Title

RJ206.M56 2002   613.2'083
                                                    QBI02-20022

Published by: Vital Health Publishing
                     P.O. Box 152
                     Ridgefield, CT 06877

For Jimmy, Eli, Dominic

and children and grandchildren
everywhere . . . they are our
hope for tomorrow.

ACKNOWLEDGEMENTS:

Many thanks to my former intern, Suzanne Shapiro, for her research of the Sports Nutrition Chapter and other book related jobs.

I would like to show great appreciation to my mentors and colleagues of the last 30 years: Robert Mendelsohn, M.D., the physicians of Homefirst Health Services, Melvyn Werbach, M.D., Jeffrey Bland, Ph.D., Robert Boxer, M.D., Liselotte Schuster, D.C., Patrick Quillin, Ph.D., R.D., Anne Louise Gittleman, M.S., Russell Blaylock, M.D., Leo Galland, M.D., Samuel Epstein, M.D., and the instructors at The University of Illinois at Chicago School of Public Health. They taught me to research, to question health "politics," and that "miracles" can happen.

I would especially like to thank my true "miracles:" my husband, Gene; my children, Steven, Carolyn, and Michael; my daughter- and sons-in-law, Shari and Jim; my in-laws, Morton and Lillian; and my precious grandchildren, Jimmy, Eli, and Dominic. They have proven their love over and over again by believing in my work and have been living examples of the rewards derived from the hard work and perseverance needed to build optimum health.

Bonnie C. Minsky

I am extremely blessed to have special people surrounding me who have, each in their own way, shown me love, kindness, generosity, support, and encouragement. Through them I have learned about life, love and relationship. They have challenged me to be more than I ever thought I would be and to do more than I ever dreamed I could. From my heart, I deeply thank of all you, including those listed below, for sharing your love, wisdom, knowledge, and experience. May you all be blessed as profoundly as you have blessed me. Namaste.

My Honored Mentors: Dr. Greg McDonald (N.D.), Dr. Rita Bettenburg (N.D.), Dr. Daniel DeLapp (D.C., L.Ac., N.D.), Dr. Satya Ambrose (N.D., L.Ac.), Dr. Karen Frangos (P.T., N.D.), Dr. Paula Crone (D.O.), Dr. Marlane Bassett (N.D.), Dr. Steven Sandberg-Lewis (N.D.), Dr. Greg Garcia (N.D.), Dr. Durr Elmore (D.C., N.D.), Dr. Virginia Osborne (N.D.), Dr. Susan Allen (N.D.), Dr. Margot Longenecker (N.D.), Dr. Laurent Chaix (N.D.), Dr. Alex Gayek (N.D.), Dr. Kevin Wilson (N.D.), Dr. Jill Stansbury (N.D.), Dr. Steve Marsden (D.V.M., N.D., L.Ac.), Dr. Rich Barrett (N.D.), Dr. Dipali Barrett (N.D.), Gayle Green, Sedrik Reavis, Shelby Royston, Maxwell Royston, Dr. Edith Taber (Ph.D.), Dr. Michael White (M.D.), Dr. Laurie Anderson (Ph.D.), Dr. Barbara Schuster (M.D.), Ansley Martin, Dr. Jonathan Wright (M.D.), Dr. Alan Gaby (M.D.), Dr. Mikael Adams (N.D.), Dr. Glen Batson (D.C.), James R. Griffith, Jean Moorehead-Libb, Sandy Papalas, Barnie Pearson, Barbara Butler and Charlie Geyer

My Friends: Dr. Shannon Grant (D.C.), Sharon Pugh, Judi Weel, Richa Eland, Kelly Garey, Bev Kleft, Carol Pater, Chris Manion, Dr. Ron and Carol Price (Ph.D.), Phil Campbell, Thomas Boddie, Enid Winters, B.J. Ruttenberg, Emil Hagopian, Dr. Sundara Delphini (N.D.), Tory Odum, Dr. Mary Galloway (N.D.), Dr. Cinda Flynn (N.D.), Eileen Hess, Mark Zamarka (J.D.), Beth Beyerl, Terr Szesny (P.A.), Kent and Erika Arett, Jan Louise Chauvin, J.J. Flentke (P.T.), Melissa Ousley, Dr. Kristin Rabai (D.C.), Dr. Bart Hodgins, (D.C.), Melanie McKee, Dr. Ann Donoghue (D.V.M.), Janette Levene, Teresa Savage, Bill Sweeney, Ron Grogg, Betty Smith, Roz McCreery, Michelle Trumfio, Deb and Rich Weaver, Lise Monet-Lunde, and special thanks to everyone, especially Gary Simms, at Chocolateer Conf ctions in Chicago for their sweet support!

My Clients and Patients: Thank you for your trust in me.

My Students: Your questions and insights impassion me. When I am with you, I am truly the student.

My Family, especially my Mother and Papa, Alva and Aldon Holk, who have graced my life with their unconditional love and devotion. I deeply appreciate and love you both. Sincere thanks to my aunt, Ellen Gross, and my uncle, Fredrick Gross, for their unending kindness and generosity and to my cousin, Dr. Linda Gross (Ph.D.) for her help with so many of my projects.

To those I hold dearly in my heart and consider to be my extended family, I thank you for your friendship. Bobbe Bermann, Nancy Bobbit, Darryn Cross, Patricia Emanuel, Dr. Sherry Gaber (D.C.), Dr. Kelly Loringer (N.D.), Ina Pinkney, Lindy Salvi, Sue Sexton, Dr. Darcy Yent (N.D., L.Ac.), Taffy and Oliver

To Jamie Alagna: Thank you for always "being there" in such a patient way!

To Dr. Diana J. White (N.D.): You are deeply loved and cherished. I thank you for your unconditional friendship for it has been one of the greatest blessings in my life. This project wouldn't have been accomplished without your help. I deeply appreciate your research and your willingness to stay up till all hours of the night to discuss ideas and outlines. Your contribution was invaluable.

To Fayne Griffiths: I immensely thank you for being a part of the most profound lessons of my life. I now understand how giving everything sometimes takes the appearance of doing and giving nothing at all.

Thanks to Frank Scott, of the Pacific College of Oriental Medicine, Rory Foster of Barat College, and Robert King, Dr. Patricia Benjamin (Ph.D.) and Chris Alvarado, of the Chicago School of Massage Therapy, for entrusting their students to me and giving me a platform upon which to do what I love the to do most . . . teach. Thanks also to Patrick Stewart for trusting his intuition!

Special thanks to Bonnie Minsky, also an honored mentor, for giving me the opportunity to be a part of this project and David Richard for his kind support of this material. It has been deeply rewarding to work with you both!

Lisa E. Holk

FOREWORD

Back in the 1960s when I was a teenager, the mantra of the new natural food movement was the statement "You are what you eat." This was a new concept in our culture, which after World War II had begun to rely on processed and artificial foods as a way to save time and effort. This resulted in a gradual change in eating habits of children across the country. Junk food, sweets and heavily processed foods became the norm. When public schools were criticized for not serving enough fresh fruit and vegetables at school lunches, the schools stated that ketchup was a vegetable, and that it was served regularly. Kids stopped bringing their lunches to school and started eating chips and soft drinks instead of good food.

Since then, the science and understanding of the role that good, clean healthy food plays in our life has increased exponentially. But at the same time, we do not seem to be taking advantage of this information. The incidence of obesity and eating disorders in children has also increased exponentially, along with illnesses like diabetes, asthma, otitis media, autism, attention deficit disorders, and a plethora of immune mediated dysfunctions caused, at least in part, by the diets our children receive. And as our children thrive, or fail to thrive, so does the health of our entire population.

So, even with the huge amount of information available to parents concerning what constitutes a healthy diet that allows their kids to mature well and be healthy, they seem to be having difficulty applying that information. Bonnie Minsky and Dr. Lisa Holk have written a book that is eminently readable and well researched, and that addresses the issue of what to feed our children in a direct and straightforward manner. They have accepted the challenge of making this wealth of information available in a practical way, so that parents can learn to understand why their children are not well, and how to rectify the situation.

The strength of this well written book lies in its direct approach, and the scientific support for the information shared. The case studies described are not rare and unusual cases: they describe children I commonly see in my practice. Drugs to treat disease are not a substitute for feeding the organism: illnesses are not a drug deficiency. But often they are the result of a nutritional deficiency. Our children are all unique: they have different needs. This book helps parents to understand what their children may need, and how to go about ensuring that they get it. The problem with nutritional information today is that there is so much of it. It can be hard to distill down to a workable diet plan. This book makes it much easier.

I recommend this book to all parents and physicians who treat children.

After all, we are what we eat.

Rita Bettenburg, N.D.
Portland, Oregon

CONTENTS

INTRODUCTION

What's wrong with our kids?

The time has finally arrived when the Western medical community is beginning to acknowledge the role of improper nutrition in the development of many of the diseases that haunt our lives today. Yet, even in light of this forward thinking, we are still participating in a mindset that allows us to ignore our bodies until they become ill. Once ill, our preoccupation and dependence on the quick fix arises and we find ourselves relying on a pill or surgery to correct a problem that appeared to "come out of nowhere." We have adopted the same "band-aid" approach for our children's health. Unfortunately, we have missed the mark. Our children are in nutritional crisis.

Did you know that:

- The incidence of childhood asthma has increased 61 percent in the United States since 1980 and the death toll from asthma has doubled in the same amount of time. Asthma affected an estimated 4.8 million U.S. children (under the age of 18 years) in 1994.
- Peanut allergy is the most common and life-threatening allergen of U.S. children.
- One out of five American children is overweight. This number has increased by more than 50 percent over the last two decades, and the number of "extremely" overweight children has nearly doubled. Overweight children are at risk for a number of health problems including heart disease, diabetes, and cancer. The Surgeon General has listed obesity as the number one public health issue of this decade.

- Research suggests that one out of every one hundred young women between ten and twenty years of age suffer from anorexia nervosa. Research also suggests that 3–4 percent of all young women and girls suffer from bulimia.

- As many as two out of five of today's teenagers risk developing osteoporosis due to lifestyle and nutritional problems.

- One out of five American children have been given a prescription for Ritalin® even though the National Institutes of Mental Health concluded that it provides no beneficial effect on academic performance, that it has, at most, an eighteen week "positive" effect on behavior and focus, that it commonly causes "cognitive toxicity," and that boys diagnosed with ADHD and treated with Ritalin® are more likely to have criminal problems in adulthood.

- The national epidemic of teen violence has ignored the widespread use of prescription antidepressant drugs among children which may be a hidden cause of violent behavior. Although safety and efficacy of Prozac® has never been tested for children, it is now routinely prescribed for children under 3 years of age (a sweet tasting liquid version is now being marketed). In fact, even the Clinton administration pushed for a reverse in the sharp rise of U.S. preschoolers being given Ritalin®, Prozac®, and other psychiatric drugs.

- Environmental and food toxins affect young children more than any other age group. Because the nervous system is particularly vulnerable to the adverse effects of toxic substances and because nerve cells normally do not regenerate once lost, it is imperative to protect our children from the damaging effects of neurotoxic substances routinely found in our air, food, and water. This is not a small undertaking when sixty-two percent of America's teenagers consume neurotoxic substances in fat-free, sugar-free, artificially colored and flavored "fake" drinks.

What has gone wrong? Why are so many of our children suffering from physical, mental, and emotional illnesses? This book is dedicated to shedding light on these questions and offering a sound approach to your child's nutritional needs from before birth through the high school years. The information in this book is based upon years of research and experience working with clients of all ages and with all types of health concerns. Many years of research and application of sound nutritional principles have proven that optimum health is directly related to preventive health measures, especially nutritional balance practiced throughout childhood. We all need to work together . . . parents, educators, and healthcare professionals to help our children reach their full potential.

AMERICA'S KIDS IN NUTRITIONAL CRISIS

≼ 1 ≽

Allergies and Food Intolerances

Did you know that asthma, allergic rhinitis, conjunctivitis and urticaria (hives) are among the most common conditions seen in the primary care physician's office today? Allergic rhinitis is responsible for approximately 9.2 million office visits to physicians yearly (CDC/HCHS, 1996). In 1996, the overall cost of allergic rhinitis totaled six billion dollars (Ray, et. al., 1999). Allergic dermatitis is the most common skin condition seen in children under 11 years of age (Lapidus, et. al., 1993). According to a study published in the *Journal of the American Medical Association (JAMA)*, the percentage of children being diagnosed annually with allergic dermatitis has increased from 3 percent to 10 percent over the last 30 years (Leung, et. al., 1997).

Allergic rhinitis is inflammation of the nasal membranes in response to an allergen. The membranes become swollen and the nose begins to "run" due to increased mucous production. Conjunctivitis is inflammation of the mucous membranes that line the eyelids. They too can become very red, watery and itchy in response to an allergen. Urticaria is a vascular reaction of the skin that produces very itchy bumps. It is commonly known as hives. All of these conditions are classic symptoms of an allergic response to a substance.

WHAT IS AN ALLERGEN?

An *allergen*, as defined in Taber's Cyclopedic Medical Dictionary, is "any substance that causes manifestations of allergy. Among common allergens are inhalants (dusts, pollens, fungi, smoke, perfumes, odors of plastics), food (wheat, eggs, milk, chocolate, strawberries), drugs

3

(aspirin, antibiotics, serums), infectious agents (bacteria, viruses, fungi, animal parasites) contactants (chemicals, animals, plants, metals) and physical agents (heat, cold, light, pressure, radiation)" (Thomas, ed., 1993). As you can see, just about anything can be an allergen. Table I lists the most common food and environmental allergens of children.

WHAT IS AN ALLERGY?

An allergy is an acquired, abnormal immune response to a substance (allergen) that does not normally cause a reaction. A normal immune system reacts by rendering an allergen inert and disposes of it by a process called phagocytosis. A hypersensitive or over-responsive immune system responds differently to an initial exposure by making antibodies to the allergen. When a susceptible child is repeatedly exposed to an allergen, the formation of an antigen-specific IgE or IgG occurs. These antibodies (proteins that signal the body that an allergen

TABLE I. MOST COMMON FOOD AND ENVIRONMENTAL ALLERGENS OF CHILDREN

Most common food allergens	Food Intolerances	Common environmental allergens
Peanuts	Yeast	Pollens
Tree nuts	Lactose	Animal dander
Cow's milk	Food dyes	Molds
Eggs	Salicylates	Grasses
Wheat	Corn	Smoke
Soy	Gluten	Chemical fumes
Fish		Dust
Shellfish		Spores
		Cockroach excretions

Sources:
American Academy of Pediatrics.
American Academy of Allergy, Asthma and Immunology.
Mahan LK and Escott-Stump S. *Krause's Food, Nutrition, & Diet Therapy.* 1996.
Rapp D., *Is This Your Child?* 1991.
United States Centers for Disease Control and Prevention. Atlanta, 1999.
United States Environmental Protection Agency. 2000.

is present) bind to mast cells. With repeated exposure to the offending allergen, these mast cells release chemical mediators such as histamine and leukotrienes into the bloodstream. These powerful mediators affect not only the target organ where the offending allergen was located but other various organs as well. The release of these powerful chemicals is what creates the reactions we see in allergic individuals. Table II lists many of the symptoms

---

TABLE II. SYMPTOMS ASSOCIATED WITH ALLERGIES.

System	Symptoms
Eyes	Itching, burning, swollen, conjunctivitis, blurred vision, photophobia (bright light causes pain), double vision, decreased night vision, allergic shiners (dark circles under the eyes thought to be caused by increased circulation to the sinuses)
Ears	Itching, Eustachian tube blockage, hearing loss, abnormal sensitivity to sound, chronic and recurrent ear infections, ringing
Nose	Itching, sneezing, *allergic salute* (upward rubbing of the nose that causes a crease mark on the nose)
Throat	Itching, difficulty swallowing, hoarse voice, excess mucous, dry mouth
Skin	Eczema (atopic dermatitis), hives (urticaria), rashes, canker sores, flushing, numbness, tingling, acne, contact dermatitis Respiratory Chest pain, shortness of breath, coughing, wheezing, coughing up blood, chronic bronchitis, asthma
Cardiovascular	Increased heart rate, arrhythmias
Gastrointestinal	Stomachache, gas/bloating, diarrhea, irritable bowel symptoms, nausea, vomiting, constipation, ulcers, weight gain, celiac disease, intestinal hemorrhage, gastritis, loss of appetite, abdominal pain
Musculoskeletal	Swelling, pain, stiffness
Genitourinary	Uncomfortable urination, increased frequency of urination, chronic bladder infection, genital itch, bedwetting
General	Headaches, migraines, chronic exhaustion, chronic infections, sinusitis
Affect	Depression, dizziness, loss of balance, mental confusion, anxiety, panic attacks, hyperactivity/behavioral problems, sleepiness, insomnia, difficulty focusing, irritability, anger, restlessness, fainting

Sources: Marz RB. *Medical Nutrition from Marz*. 1997.
Rapp D, *Is This Your Child?* 1991.
Tierney LM, McPhee SJ, Papadakis MA. *Current Medical Diagnosis & Treatment*. 2000.

associated with allergies. It is important to note that an allergy is an *acquired* hypersensitivity reaction to a substance. This means that if we, as parents, can support our child's immune system by minimizing their exposure to those foods and environmental stimuli which are likely to cause an allergic reaction, we may be able to decrease the probability that our child will develop allergies.

WHAT MAKES SOME PEOPLE SUSCEPTIBLE TO POTENTIAL ALLERGENS WHILE OTHERS HAVE NO REACTIONS?

Genetics plays an important role. A child is more likely to suffer from allergies if there is a family history of allergic disorders. How a child's immune system develops after birth has also been found to play an important role in allergic reactions. Human breast milk supplies infants with crucial immune modulators, those substances that fight off potential allergens. Health practitioners are realizing that food allergies are notably common during the first two years of life, when the gut barrier is immature and the immune system is still developing. Because a baby's immune system is not fully developed at birth, breast milk and proper introduction of foods is crucial in developing and maintaining a child's digestion and immune system. Up to five percent of children today have food allergies compared to one to two percent in adults.

Many more children suffer from food intolerances, such as gluten or lactose intolerance. If you are an expectant mom, or currently breastfeeding, remember that it is recommended that you do not introduce your baby to solid foods before the age of six months. If you have a family history of food allergies or intolerances, wait two weeks between introducing each new food in the following order: rice, banana, pear, carrot, squash, sweet potato, barley, green beans, applesauce, oats, peas, egg yolk, turkey, and chicken. At one year of age, dairy products may be introduced, beginning with butter.

DIAGNOSING ALLERGIES

Allergy symptoms can occur immediately after exposure to an offending substance or may take many days to manifest. Because of the great variations in severity and timing, allergies are one of the most frustrating ailments to diagnose. Many classically trained physicians will only diagnose that an allergy is present when there is an immune response that produces the antigen-specific IgE or IgG. However, not all people who present with the signs and symptoms of *allergy* actually produce these immunoglobulins. When this occurs, we refer to an individual as having an *intolerance*. Food and environmental intolerances can cause symptoms that are just as severe and debilitating as those seen in an IgE mediated allergy.

To detect if an allergy is present, physicians will either test your child's blood to see if any immunoglobulins such as IgE are present or they will introduce an allergen into your child's skin to see if a physical reaction occurs. If a physical reaction occurs such as a welt or wheal (raised, red area), then it is suspected that the child may have immunoglobulins in their blood and further testing is done. These testing methods are most sensitive and specific for inhalant and stinging insect sensitivities. Frequent false positive results occur when testing for food allergies because the testing materials are not very pure. As a general rule, cow's milk, egg, peanut, tree nuts, soy, and wheat account for about 90 percent confirmed allergies in young children. All positive food test results should be correlated with clinical history and should be confirmed with repeated challenge tests.

In addition to clinical tests, a thorough physical exam can offer many clues to the diagnosis of allergy. Some of the physical signs often seen include:

- "allergic shiners" (dark circles under the eyes)
- eyelid swelling
- redness of the eyes
- cobblestoning of the throat (rough looking patterns in the back of the throat from lymphatic swelling)

- creases on the surface of the nose from the child constantly rubbing/pushing their nose up toward their forehead (often called the "allergic salute")
- abnormal lung sounds
- an increased heart/pulse rate evident after ingestion of a reactive food

The importance of a thorough exam cannot be stressed enough. Should you suspect that your child is suffering from allergies or intolerances, seek the diagnostic skills of a licensed health professional who has had extensive experience with allergies and intolerances. Also recognize that there are other pathologies that can imitate allergies.

THE GREAT IMITATORS

Many parents become discouraged when they suspect that their child is allergic, but traditional tests show negative for antibody responses. In these cases, your child is probably suffering from a food sensitivity or intolerance. Because the symptoms are very similar to allergy responses, we call food intolerances "the great imitators."

CANDIDIASIS

Candidiasis is a complex medical syndrome characterized by an overgrowth in the gastrointestinal tract of the usually benign yeast *candida albicans*. Candidiasis can affect many systems in the body including the gastrointestinal, genitourinary, endocrine, nervous and immune systems. *Candida albicans* lives harmoniously in the digestive and vaginal tracts. If the normal lining of the intestinal tract is damaged, or if the immune system is weakened, the body can absorb yeast cells, yeast particles and various toxins excreted by the yeast. Yeast overgrowth may also occur when normal gut flora becomes unbalanced. The most common cause of candidiasis in children is the overuse of antibiotics. The use of steroid and cortisone-like drugs may also predispose a child to this syndrome (see Chapter 3: Immune System Dysfunction).

If your child is showing any of the following symptoms, yeast overgrowth may be the problem:

- Fatigue, drowsiness
- Irritability, mood swings
- Depression
- Headache
- Muscle pain
- Skin problems such as rashes and chronic itching
- Digestive disturbances including stomach aches, gas, bloating, constipation and/or diarrhea, mucous in stools
- Poor memory, inability to concentrate
- Nasal itching and/or congestion
- Wheezing, shortness of breath, chest tightness, cough
- Chronic, recurrent infections
- Ear aches, hearing loss

Diagnosis of this condition is often made based on a complete history, a blood test for Candida antigens, or scoring high on a written Candida questionnaire. Some physicians will order a comprehensive stool and digestive analysis (CDSA) which detects the presence of candida and gives useful information about many factors that play an important role in the general well-being of the gut.

CELIAC DISEASE (CELIAC SPRUE, GLUTEN-SENSITIVE ENTEROPATHY, NON-TROPICAL SPRUE)

Celiac disease, another great imitator of allergies, is a genetic chronic intestinal malabsorption disorder caused by intolerance to gluten. Gluten, which is found primarily in grains such as wheat, barley, rye, spelt, oats, and millet, is the "glue" that holds grains together. When the gluten cannot be absorbed, the villi on the intestinal surface are destroyed, resulting in a loss of absorptive area. Removal of the gluten from the diet allows for the regeneration of the intestinal surface. Symptoms of this disease usually appear in the first three years of life once cereals are introduced into the diet, but it may take years before a proper diagnosis is made.

Symptoms of gluten intolerance include:

- Weight loss or inability to gain weight
- Poor growth
- Malnutrition from the impaired absorption of protein, fat, and fat-soluble vitamins and minerals
- Gas and bloating
- Weakness and fatigue
- Foul-smelling, fatty bowel movements (often yellowish in color)
- Anemia
- A tendency toward bruising and easy bleeding
- Bone pain, skeletal deformities
- Muscle pain and spasm
- Numbness and tingling of the hands and feet

Since the complications of this disease can be dramatic, it is important to have any child that has difficulty digesting grains tested as soon as possible. Diagnosis of this condition is based upon a thorough history, physical exam and lab work. Since this disease causes malabsorption, identifying and correcting any nutritional deficiencies is extremely important as is removing all gluten from the diet. Besides ordering blood work to evaluate for nutritional deficiencies, your physician may request gastrointestinal barium studies and a tissue biopsy before assigning a diagnosis.

People of Irish and Scottish descent are particularly prone to this genetic disorder. In the United Kingdom, gluten intolerance is often diagnosed within the first few months after the presentation of symptoms. In the United States, it typically takes up to **eight years** for a diagnosis to be made.

An excellent magazine is available for those who suffer from any kind of allergy, intolerance or sensitivity. *Sully's Living Without* is a lifestyle guide full of ideas about lifestyle changes and fantastic recipes for any type of food restriction. The magazine addresses a wide variety of health issues including "allergies, food sensitivities, multiple chemical sensitivities, wheat intolerance, gluten intolerance, lactose intolerance, dairy allergies, eating disorders, asthma, diabetes, dermatitis, gastroenterology-related disorders, diets that heal, celiac disease, anaphylaxis and the common allergens of egg, dairy, wheat, peanuts, tree nuts, shellfish, fish, corn, soy and gluten" (*Sully's Living Without*, 2001). Visit their website, www.LivingWithout.com or call (630) 415-3378 to subscribe.

WEAK DIGESTIVE ENZYMES

Weak digestive enzymes interfere with the proper digestion of food and, therefore, allow the passage of larger undigested food particles into the gut. It is theorized that these larger molecules make their way through a compromised gut into the bloodstream where they are "attacked" by the immune system. The immune system will not react to properly digested food particles, as they are too small to be recognized by the immune system. Therefore, if you notice undigested food in your child's stool on a regular basis, it may be helpful to give your child digestive enzymes to enhance their digestive ability. Chewable bromelain (found naturally in pineapple) and papain (found naturally in papaya) are mild and often powerful enough to correct the problem.

ALLERGY/FOOD INTOLERANCE TREATMENTS

Many treatment protocols, conventional and alternative, offer relief of symptoms but may not address the underlying cause of symptoms. Make sure your health practitioner looks for the cause of your child's symptoms so that the treatment plan can be designed to re-establish homeostasis in the body. Be cautious about using medicines that merely treat your child's symptoms. These medicines can actually be suppressive and interfere with your child's innate ability to heal.

There are select vitamins, minerals, and flavonoids that can help your child on their road to recovery. A short list is provided here with brief explanations as to their mechanisms of action. Your health care practitioner can guide you as to the use and proper dosage of these valuable tools.

- **Vitamin C** is an excellent, potent antioxidant which helps stabilize the immune system. It inhibits histamines thereby helping to reduce inflammation. It improves adrenal function, which can be overtaxed in allergic, inflammatory conditions.

- **Vitamin B$_6$** is extremely important in the proper functioning of the immune system. It is necessary for the production of antibodies, red blood cells and hydrochloric acid in the stomach (a powerful stomach acid necessary for proper digestion in the gut). It is an important co-factor that works with more than 60 different enzymes in the body. It is also important in strengthening adrenal function.

- **Vitamin E**, an immune system stabilizer, interacts extensively with other antioxidant nutrients, especially vitamin C and selenium. It supports gastrointestinal health and has strong anti-inflammatory properties.

- **Quercetin**, a non-citrus bioflavonoid, has demonstrated significant anti-inflammatory activity in the body. In addition to possessing antioxidant qualities, it helps to increase vitamin C uptake in cells. Because of its ability to inhibit the manufacture and release of histamine and other allergic/inflammatory mediators, it is commonly used to support the treatment of asthma and allergies.

- **Magnesium** plays a critical role in many enzymatic and cellular functions. It promotes relaxation of the bronchial smooth muscles making breathing easier. It is used clinically in emergency situations to halt acute asthma attacks. Magnesium interacts extensively with other minerals, especially B$_6$. Low magnesium levels are suspected in patients with chronic allergies and/or food intolerances.

STEPS TO TAKE IF YOU SUSPECT YOUR CHILD HAS ALLERGIES/INTOLERANCES

1. Begin by keeping a symptom/food diary. Try to identify the foods or environmental stimuli to which your child may be reacting. Take this information with you when you see your health practitioner.

2. Avoid all heavily refined foods, preservatives, food dyes, artificial food additives, and toxic household products. All of these, singly or cumulatively, can harm your child's immune system. (See Chapters 11 and 13 for steps to avoid harmful products.)

3. If you suspect allergies, instead of intolerances, seek help from a board-certified allergist. This specially trained physician will be able to do a complete work-up and determine if there is an overt allergy that produces an immunoglobulin response.

4. If you suspect the possibility of celiac disease, notify your child's physician so the appropriate testing will be done. A referral to a gastroenterologist may also be necessary.

5. If allergies have been ruled out, there is a great possibility that your child is dealing with an intolerance or a yeast overgrowth. You can use the elimination diet (see Chapter 13 for details to determine any intolerances that may be present).

6. If your child is dealing with a yeast overgrowth, seek a qualified practitioner who is adept at determining what kind of supplementation will be beneficial. Some children may improve with the addition of digestive enzymes and probiotics, such as lactobacillus acidophilus. Re-establishing a balanced gut flora takes time. Strict adherence to a yeast-free diet is an essential part of the therapy (see Chapter 13 for details).

Personal Case Study #1

A breast-feeding mother brought in her five-month-old daughter, Geraldine, because the infant suffered from full body eczema and constant spitting-up. Geraldine was exclusively breast-fed. Allergy testing had revealed no common food allergens. The pediatrician had recommended that she switch Geraldine from breast-feeding to a low allergy infant formula. I urged the mother to try the two-week elimination diet first, to use allergy-free detergent for anything that would touch Geraldine's skin, and to add baking soda in the rinse cycle when washing her clothes to neutralize toxins.

The results were dramatic. Although Geraldine's mother went through a tired, headachy withdrawal period for five days, Geraldine stopped spitting-up immediately and was free of eczema in nine days. The triggers were blue detergent, corn (the mother's favorite nightly snack had been popcorn), and salicylates, especially the mother's morning orange juice and nightly salad of balsamic vinegar and tomatoes.

Geraldine's mother was relieved by Geraldine's rapid recovery, but even more impressed that her twenty extra pounds that she assumed was "baby weight" came off rapidly and her daily low-grade chronic headaches and stomachaches disappeared.

We added new foods and drinks very slowly when Geraldine started eating table foods to prevent or minimize food sensitivities. Today, at age three, Geraldine can eat any dye-free, nitrate-free foods without having a reaction.

DR. HOLK'S RX

Homeopathy has been shown to be effective in the alleviation of acute allergies. The following remedies are commonly used. Choosing the right remedy can be tricky. The following are given only as guidelines. Match the symptoms your child is experiencing as closely as you can to one of the symptom pictures stated below. If at first you don't succeed, try again. A homeopathic practitioner can be invaluable for helping your child to abate asthma and allergy problems. To find a qualified practitioner in your area contact any of the organizations listed at the end of this chapter.

REMEDY	SYMPTOM PICTURE
Allium Cepa	Stinging nasal discharge with possible chapping and /or sores around the nose or on the upper lip. The nose runs "like a faucet" and the child may stuff tissue in their nose to stop it from running. Eyes water profusely. The child may seek open air and cool rooms and may avoid warm rooms. The symptoms may begin or be more pronounced on the left side. The child may be sensitive to light.
Arsenicum Album	This nasal discharge is also stinging but here we see dripping from a nose that is swollen and difficult or impossible to breathe through. Eyes burn. The child may be very sensitive to light. The symptoms may begin or be more pronounced on the right side. The child will often feel better with his head elevated and with external heat applications.
Euphrasia	This remedy focuses on the eyes instead of the nose. Use it if the eyes seem to be most bothersome to the child. The eyes will be inflamed and extremely irritated often with a thick, burning, yellowish discharge. They will itch and/or burn. There may be profuse nasal discharge. The child may feel worse in the morning and get better as the day progresses into night. The child may have a constant, tickling cough that improves when lying down and as the day goes by.
Natrum Muriaticum	This remedy is often used for chronic hayfever-type symptoms, especially in children who have a tendency to be somewhat intellectual. They may have a nasal discharge that appears white. Their symptoms often get worse when they are in warm rooms. They may prefer open air, cool bathing and lying on their right side when resting.
Nux Vomica	Here you will see intense sneezing and nasal congestion upon waking in the morning. These children tend to be profusely discharging in the morning and during the day but then "dry up" in the evening. These children will seek warmth because it improves their condition and allows them to breathe through their nose more freely. They may even prefer warm drinks.
Pulsatilla	This remedy is often used for the symptoms of hayfever. The child will present with very itchy eyes and a watery discharge from the nose. They improve with cold applications and chose to be in air-conditioned areas. Overheating makes them feel worse.

Sabadilla	Use this when your child is sneezing constantly especially if the sneezing produces tearing. The sneezing will intensify when the child comes in contact with anything that is cold but will improve when coming into contact with anything that is warm. There will be a profuse watery nasal discharge and the nose may be very itchy or it may be stuffed. The nose tends to tickle and/or itch. The eyes will water in open air and bright lights. Cold tends to make them feel worse.

SOURCES: Kruzel T. *The Homeopathic Emergency Guide.* 1992.
Vermeulen F. *Concordant Materia Medica.* 1997.
Weintraub S. *Allergies and Holistic Healing.* 1997.

To find a qualified homeopathic practitioner in your area contact:

American Institute of Homeopathy
801 N. Fairfax Street, Suite 306
Alexandria, Virginia 22314
Phone: (888) 445-9988
Website: www.homeopathyusa.org

Council for Homeopathic Certification
1060 North 4th Street
San Jose, CA 95112
Phone: (408) 971-5915

Homeopathic Academy of Naturopathic Physicians
12132 S.E. Foster Place
Portland, OR 97266
Phone: (503) 761-3298
Website: www.healthy.net/hanp

North American Society of Homeopaths
1122 East Pike Street, # 1122
Seattle, WA 98122
Phone: (206) 720-7000
Website: www.homeopathy.org

For more information on food allergies and intolerances:

The Food Allergy and Anaphylaxis Network (FAAN)
10400 Eaton Place, Suite 107
Fairfax, Virginia 22030-2208
Phone: (800) 929-4040
Website: www.foodallergy.org

National Institute of Allergy and Infectious Diseases (NIAID)
Office of Communications and Public Liaison
Building 31, Room 7A-50
31 Center Drive MSC 2520
Bethesda, Maryland 20892-2520
Website: www.niaid.nih.gov

FAUS (Feingold Association of the United States)
P.O. Box 6550
Alexandria, VA 22306
Phone: (800) 321-FAUS
Website: www.feingold.org

Sully's *Living Without*, Inc.
P.O. Box 132
Clarendon Hills, IL 60514-0132
Phone: (630) 415-3378
Website: www.LivingWithout.com

ᢂ 2 ᢓ

Asthma

To breathe or not to breathe is the question for over 17 million Americans, 4.8 million of whom are children under the age of 18 years (United States Centers for Disease Control, 1998; ATS Update, 1998). According to Dr. Gary Rachelefsky, past president of the Academy of Allergy, Asthma and Immunology (AAAAI), "the prevalence and impact of asthma has exploded." From 1980 to 1994, the prevalence of asthma increased by 75 percent (United States Centers for Disease Control, 1998). In 1997, the National Institute of Allergy and Infectious Disease reported that asthmatic children missed more than 10 million school days annually (United States NIAID, 1997). The cost of this disease is high. Statistics from the American Lung Association reveal health care costs for asthma in the United States alone total more than $9.8 billion annually (American Lung Association, 1998).

WHAT IS ASTHMA?

Asthma is a reactive inflammatory airway disorder that occurs in response to an internal or external stimulus. It is characterized by episodes of shortness of breath, chest tightness, wheezing and coughing which may be relieved spontaneously or as a result of therapy.

Two general types of asthma are recognized based on the stimulus that provokes the attack. Extrinsic asthma has a genetic tendency and is the most common form of the disease. Onset often occurs before the age of ten years with twice as many boys being affected as girls. This form is considered to be an "allergic" form and is often accompanied by other hereditary allergies such as hives, allergic

19

rhinitis, and eczema. Intrinsic or idiosyncratic asthma is often the result of exposure to an upper respiratory infection, chemical irritants found in the environment or certain drugs such as aspirin. Many asthmatics have a mixed type of asthma that is triggered by stimuli in either category. Table I illustrates common intrinsic and extrinsic triggers.

DIAGNOSIS AND MEDICATIONS

The diagnosis of asthma is best made by a physician who will order and evaluate a series of pulmonary function tests. These tests measure the volume of the lungs as well as the amount of air that can be expired. Since asthma is characterized by reversible airway obstruction, evaluation

---

TABLE I. COMMON TRIGGERS FOR ASTHMA

Extrinsic Triggers	Intrinsic Triggers
Pollen	Respiratory tract infections
Animal dander, saliva and urine	Drugs, i.e., aspirin, beta-adrenergic antagonists
Household dust	Fatigue
Dust mites	Stress
Cockroach feces and saliva	Endocrine changes
Molds	Variations in temperature and humidity
Feather pillows	Coughing or laughing
Smoke	Exercise
Air pollution, ozone	Gastroesophageal Reflux Disease (GERD)
Exposure to chemicals fumes, i.e., common fuels, natural gas, fuel oil, kerosene, wood, coal	
Food additives, coloring agents, sulfiting agents	
Unrecognized food sensitivities and/or allergies	
Centrally heated homes	

SOURCES:
Fauci AS, Braunwald E, Isselbacher KJ, et. al. *Harrison's Principles of Internal Medicine Companion Handbook,* 14th ed., New York: McGraw-Hill, 1998. p. 722.
United States Environmental Protection Agency

is often done before and after the administration of a short-acting bronchodilator to see if the airways respond to such stimulation. It is highly recommended that asthmatic children learn to use an expiratory peak flow meter to monitor their breathing. It is a hand-held device that can help to alert a child to airway restriction before it becomes severe.

Despite the improved protocols for treatment, death rates from asthma, although still low, continue to rise. The cause is not clear. Since many asthma drugs used have severe side effects, and some can actually potentiate the asthma when overused, there is concern that these drugs may play a role in the increased death rate (Spitzer, WO, et. al., 1992; Meier, CR and Jick, H., 1997). It is, therefore, imperative that parents and children understand the purpose and correct use of each medication prescribed. It is also imperative to monitor the number of times your child is taking medication each day in order to evaluate the overall effectiveness of the treatment protocol.

Corticosteriods used to reduce inflammation actually decrease the ability of the immune system to respond to an invader, therefore, increasing the risk of infection. Long-term systemic doses have been shown to cause osteoporosis, increased appetite, weight gain, weakened connective tissue, swelling, hypertension, peptic ulcers and mood disorders. Inhaled corticosteroids can reduced the need for systemic corticosteroid treatment but also carry the risk of oral yeast infections. Given that up to 90 percent of the drug is actually swallowed and goes into the GI tract, candidiasis of the mouth and throat, often referred to as thrush, can occur. Make sure your child rinses his mouth after each administration to reduce the possibility of a thrush infection. A spacer can also be used with the drug canister. A spacer reduces the amount of drug that gets deposited in the mouth. Since corticosteriods have no direct effect on the lung but instead affect the cells involved with the inflammatory process, they should never be relied upon for quick relief of an acute asthma attack.

Mast cell stabilizers work to inhibit mast cells from releasing their chemical mediators that cause increased vascular permeability, bronchial spasm, and local inflammation. This response is called an **immediate hypersensitivity** response and in its most severe form is referred to as **anaphylaxis.** These drugs are often best used with those who have seasonal asthma where the trigger has been identified. These drugs are not to be relied upon for quick relief of an asthma attack but are used preventively to reduce airway reactivity.

Allergy injections remain somewhat controversial on the alternative side of the coin but are well accepted in allopathic medicine. A small amount of allergen is administered to the patient over a period of time with hopes that the patient will become desensitized to that allergen and, therefore, not react to it when it is encountered in the environment. The theory certainly seems valid but, in reality, this approach can create a chronic low-grade inflammatory state that may actually keep the child ill and rundown.

Bronchodilators (albuterol, epinephrine [given subcutaneously], terbutaline, metaproterenol sulfate and others) are medications that stimulate the sympathetic nervous system producing relaxation of the spasmed smooth muscles in the bronchi. Side effects of these medications include tremors, headaches, dizziness, cardiac palpitations and arrhythmias, and decreased concentration. Bronchodilators are used to control chronic asthma as well as to abate an acute asthma attack. Because of the potency of these medications, it is important to understand how much of the drug can be administered without overdosing. Asthma is a life-threatening condition that requires constant monitoring.

A child who is taking asthma medications may be irritable, easily fatigued, overly sensitive, and constantly anxious. It is important to notify all individuals engaged with your child, especially teachers, about your child's condition. Educate them about the side effects of the drugs and what to do in the case of an emergency. At home, make allowances for their increased sensitivity by supporting them with a calm and loving environment.

NEW RESEARCH SHOWS A CONNECTION BETWEEN ANTIBIOTIC USE AND ASTHMA

A study published in the *Journal of Clinical and Experimental Allergy* found that children given an antibiotic during the first year of life were four times as likely to develop asthma symptoms than children who had not received antibiotics. Professor Crane, co-researcher of this study, noted that, *Broad spectrum antibiotics came into clinical usage in the 1960s, and their use coincides with the time trends for the increasing prevalence of asthma. There is a plausible mechanism, namely that broad-spectrum antibiotics may alter and reduce bowel flora and thus switch off the immunological signals that these gut bacteria send to the developing immune system* (Wickens K, et. al., 1999). Table II summarizes the results of their study.

Why is there an increase in the number of asthmatic cases despite improved medications?

Theories abound as to why the number of diagnosed cases has dramatically increased over the past two decades. As stated, some believe that the overuse of medications may be to blame. Others cite increased air pollution and exposure to allergens found in the home. What may also be a factor is the increased reliance, especially over the over the past two decades, on frozen convenience and "junk" foods, both of which have little nutritional value and are packed with food additives. Scientists in the United Kingdom and Saudi Arabia compared 114 children with a history of asthma to 202 non-asthmatic children and found that those children with the lowest intake of vegetables, vitamin E, and minerals were more likely to suffer from the disease. The study abstract notes that these findings are consistent with previous studies in adults and supports the hypothesis that diet plays a major role in the increases of asthma and allergies seen worldwide (Hijazi N, et. al., 2000).

TABLE II. INCREASED ODDS RATIO OF A CHILD DEVELOPING ASTHMA with the use of antibiotics

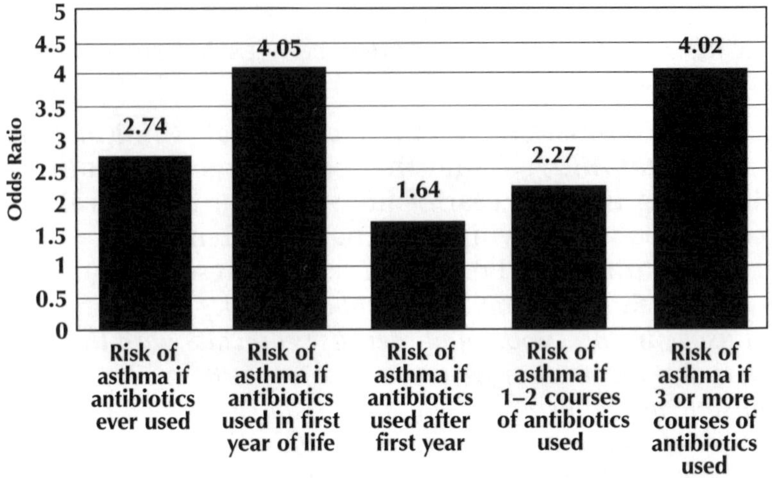

	Odds Ratio

The following chart shows Odds Ratio (y-axis, 0 to 5):

- Risk of asthma if antibiotics ever used: 2.74
- Risk of asthma if antibiotics used in first year of life: 4.05
- Risk of asthma if antibiotics used after first year: 1.64
- Risk of asthma if 1–2 courses of antibiotics used: 2.27
- Risk of asthma if 3 or more courses of antibiotics used: 4.02

Wickens K, Pearce N, Crane J, Beasley R. Journal of Clinical and Experimental Allergy. 29:766-771, 1999

THE MILK DEBATE

In 1979, Kokkonen and his colleagues studied the level of stomach acid secretion in infants with cow's milk intolerance. After giving the infants a single dose of cow's milk they found the maximal secretion to be one-third of the amount that healthy infants produced. These infants were then treated with human or soy milk and the maximal level of stomach acid returned to normal but took six months to do so (Kokkonen J, et. al., 1979).

In another study, ten-year-old subjects who had manifested cow's milk allergy before the age of one year were evaluated for ongoing allergies and other atopic phenomenon. Of the 56 children examined, all but four had become tolerant to a small amount of milk protein but when a larger amount was given, approximately 45 percent reported digestive disturbances. The incidence of asthma, allergies, recurrent ear infections and skin disorders were three to four times more likely in this group. (Tikkanen S, et. al., 2000).

Recurrent ear infections have also been positively correlated with cow's milk allergy. In 1999, a study of 56 milk-allergic children found that children with cow's milk allergy in infancy, even when properly treated, had many more episodes of recurrent ear infections. Ear infections were also more likely to occur in children who had asthma and allergic rhinitis (inflammation of the nasal mucosa) (Juntti H, et. al., 1999).

Human breast milk, however, has been associated with a lower incidence of asthma symptoms. A study of 2,834 Australian children done by Dr.Wendy Oddy, MPH, of TVW Telethon Institute for Child Health in West Perth, Western Australia, found that children who were given a form of milk other than their mother's milk in the first four months of their life were 27 percent more likely to have doctor-diagnosed asthma by age six and 41 percent more likely to have wheezed in the past 12 months (American Lung Association/American Thoracic Society International Conference, April, 1999).

Human mother's breast milk is perfect nutrition for the newborn and young infant. Breast-feeding supplies molecules that are important components and activators of the infant's immune system. Breast-feeding is especially crucial at birth because an infant's immune and digestive systems are immature. These systems rely on the nutrients, proteins, carbohydrates, fats, antibodies, enzymes and hormones supplied in the mother's milk for growth and protection. Colostrum, the sticky yellowish fluid high in protein that is delivered to the infant with its first suckling, confers important immune factors, cleansing the baby's intestinal tract and ridding the body of mucus. After the colostrum is utilized, breast milk, a thin white, bluish liquid, supplies the perfect combination of vitamins, minerals, fats, proteins and carbohydrates. Human breast milk aids the development of healthy flora in the intestine and helps with absorption of essential minerals like calcium and magnesium (Zand J, et. al., 1994). Breastfed children have a lower incidence of ear infections, food allergies, gastrointestinal disturbances and constipation (Schwartz MW, et. al., 1997).

Clinical allergy researchers, well aware of the global rise of asthma and allergies, recommend breastfeeding in infancy. Human breast milk is crucial for the normal development of the immune and digestive systems. Problems can arise, however, when allergens, pathogens, or toxins are transferred through the milk. An infant may have a predisposition to allergies and be reacting to something that the mother is eating. When this occurs, it is necessary to put the mother on an elimination diet and observe the response of the infant (see Chapter 13 for further details).

COULD ANYTHING ELSE BE GOING ON?

More and more research is showing that a possible etiology for asthma is a defect in the gut/mucus membranes that causes increased permeability. For whatever reason, asthmatic children seem to have a predisposition to gastrointestinal problems that express themselves in a number of ways, including hypochlorhydria (low stomach acid levels), possible malabsorption syndromes, and acid balance disturbances. These gastrointestinal problems promote the retention of carbon dioxide and make breathing more difficult. Since the gut offers one of the first lines of defense against attack by invaders, any disturbance in the integrity of the gut tissues can cause a maladapted immune response resulting in an increased number of infections and a chronic level of low-grade inflammation.

THREE THINGS YOU CAN DO TO HELP CONTROL ASTHMA

FIRST, REMOVE THE TRIGGERS.

Many or all of the triggers associated with asthma may be affecting your child. Keeping track of your child's symptoms and associating the symptoms with the event that triggered the attack will give you guidance as to what modifications need to be made. The United States Environmental Protection Agency has a wonderful website (*www.epa.gov*) that offers practical information for dealing with dander, molds, combustion pollutants, cockroaches, dust mites, ozone, house dust and secondhand smoke. Also see the Appendix for a list of non-toxic household products.

Food sensitivities and allergies can be a little more difficult to determine, especially when reactions can be delayed many hours. The best way to evaluate food sensitivities is to put your child on a diet that eliminates the most common food allergens for a period of time. The suspected allergen/food is then reintroduced into the diet and the child is observed for a reaction. The standard elimination diet removes the most common food allergens which includes dairy products, wheat, corn, soy, eggs, peanuts, nuts, shellfish, salicylates and food additives, including MSG, for two weeks (see Chapter 13 for details regarding the application of the Elimination Diet).

I also recommend seeing an allergist or other physician who is an expert in environmental toxins. Contact the American Preventive Medicine Association (*www.apma.net*) for names of doctors in your area.

SECOND, SUPPORT THE BODY WITH PROPER NUTRITION.

The more nutrient-dense the food, the more health benefits your child will receive. Add foods rich in omega-3 fatty acids such as walnuts, pumpkin seeds, flax seed oil, salmon, tuna, mackerel, and cold water fish to help inhibit a biochemical pathway that promotes inflammation. Limit the consumption of red meats and dairy products that contain arachadonic acid and, therefore, promote the same inflammatory pathway. Increase the consumption of foods rich in bioflavonoids, especially high quercetin foods, because they have been shown to help stabilize mast cells by making them less likely to release their contents which initiate inflammation.

Onions, apples, kale, green beans, sweet cherries, and grape skins are high in quercetin. Avoid excess calcium and limit bananas because they can actually potentiate the inflammatory pathway. Increase the consumption of foods high in magnesium such as fatty fish, dark green vegetables, avocado, pumpkin seeds and blackstrap molasses. Eliminate foods containing MSG, sulfites, food colorings, white sugar and artificial sweeteners.

THIRD, SUPPORT WITH USEFUL SUPPLEMENTATION.

I always recommend the following supplements to my asthmatic clients. The dosages will vary depending upon your child's age and body weight, so it is best to see a qualified health professional before implementing any of the following into your child's protocol.

Vitamin B$_6$ (Pyridoxine): Pyridoxine is required for many of the chemical reactions that occur in the body and is essential for the formation of neurotransmitters and the protective myelin sheaths that surround nerves. It is also involved in the synthesis of intrinsic factor, which is a substance normally found in gastric juice that makes absorption of B$_{12}$ possible.

Russell Marz, ND, believes that people are not even getting the RDI (recommended dietary intakes) for B$_6$ because so many things in our environment are antagonistic to its absorption. Dr. Blaylock, a neurosurgeon, agrees. Table III identifies the most common B$_6$ antagonists.

Vitamin B$_{12}$: The substantiation for using vitamin B$_{12}$ is anectodal. Many doctors of naturopathic medicine include this in their treatment protocol for asthma. Jonathan Wright, MD, supports its use and finds it to be especially effective for sulfite-sensitive asthmatics. Intramuscular injections are the administration route of choice. Asthmatics may have a tendency to be B$_{12}$ deficient given that many are hypochlorhydric. The same cells in the stomach which secrete gastric acid also secrete

TABLE III. ANTAGONISTS TO VITAMIN B_6 (PYRIDOXINE)

Hydrazine compounds such as those in medications (isonicoyinic acid hydrazine and Hydralazine, a blood pressure medication) and hydralazine in store bought mushrooms

Antioxidants used in the petroleum industry

Food dyes: Tartrazine (yellow dye #5) and caramel color

Oxidized and hydrogenated fats found in our food supply such as barbecued and fried foods, most potato and corn chips, commercial margarines, shortenings, etc.

Birth Control Pills

Penicillamine and cycloserine

Environmental toxins such as fuel fumes and tobacco smoke

Alcohol

Monosodium glutamate and Aspartame

Sources:

Marz RB. *Medical Nutrition from Marz.* 2nd ed. Portland, Oregon: Omni-Press. 1997.
Blaylock R. *Excitotoxins: The Taste That Kills,* Santa Fe, New Mexico: Health Press, 1994.

the intrinsic factor needed for vitamin B_{12} absorption in the small intestine.

Vitamin C: Vitamin C is the main antioxidant found in the fluid lining of the lungs. The constant tissue destruction that occurs with the inflammation of asthma, resulting in the release of free radicals, places a high burden upon the antioxidants found there.

Studies have shown that asthmatics tend to have low levels of intracellular vitamin C and that their blood levels are inversely correlated with the degree of wheezing. It is theorized that vitamin C may be protective for asthmatics due to its ability to lower blood histamine levels and decrease bronchospasm.

Vitamin C also works synergistically with vitamin E, another potent antioxidant, by reactivating the vitamin E in the body so it can continue to play its role as an antioxidant. Since many asthmatics have an acid imbalance, it is recommended that non-acidic or buffered forms of vitamin C be used. Vitamin C derived from sago palm or Ester C with added calcium and magnesium are my recommendations.

Vitamin E: Insufficient intake of vitamin E has also been linked to an increased risk of bronchial asthma. Vitamin E plays a synergistic role with vitamin C. Since current studies support that asthmatics have lower levels of free radical scavengers, supplementation with antioxidants may play an important role in the modulation of inflammation (Shanmugasundaram KR, et. al., 2001).

Magnesium: Studies show that asthmatics also tend to have significantly lower intercellular levels of magnesium. Magnesium plays an important role in over 300 chemical reactions that occur in the body. It relaxes smooth muscles around the airways, therefore reducing bronchoconstriction. It also reduces airway inflammation by stabilizing mast cells. One's intake of magnesium has also been inversely related to the severity of the symptoms in asthma. Many emergency rooms are now using intravenous magnesium to abate an acute asthma attack.

Molybdenum: Jonathan Wright, MD, has also correlated sulfite sensitivities with a possible molybdenum deficiency and has found that intravenous administration of molybdenum substantially decreases the sensitivity. To find out if your child is sulfite sensitive, a urine dipstick test can be done to detect if sulfites are present. They should not be.

Quercetin: Quercetin is a non-citrus bioflavinoid with potent anti-inflammatory, antiviral, and antioxidant properties. Taken in pill form, it has a greater potency than from foods. It has been shown to inhibit the breakdown of mast cells and, therefore, block the release of inflammatory agents. Its action can be potentiated by taking bromelain (naturally occurring in pineapple) at the same time. It may take four to six weeks before the effects of quercetin become evident.

Dr. Holk's Case Study #2

Serge was an eight-year-old boy who was suffering terribly with his asthma. He had been diagnosed with the disease at the age of four years. His asthma woke him every night. At his worst, he was visiting the emergency room 2–3 times each week. The albuterol and corticosteriod inhalers he was using were ineffective. He was napping 2–3 hours each day and complained constantly of stomachaches. He was later put on a nebulizer and told to use it as needed. By the time I saw him he was using the nebulizer every 4–6 hours with very little improvement.

The first step in the treatment of asthma is always to identify and remove the offending allergens. In Serge's case, he had to eliminate all dairy products, tomatoes, peanuts, mixed nuts, white sugar, molasses, cocoa, sugar substitutes, MSG, and all food preservatives.

His environment was modified by removing all triggers and placing non-allergenic covers over his mattress and pillowcases. An air filter was added to his room.

Since Serge was not willing to swallow pills, we compromised in giving him a chewable multivitamin and a chewable vitamin C tablet. I did not want him to have the fructose or corn syrup in the tablets but felt that getting the vitamins and minerals into him was essential. We also gave him a high potency powdered form of acidophilus which he took two times a day before meals.

Serge's family ate out a lot. Serge loved hamburgers and would eat them whenever he could. Red meat tends to produce arachodonic acid in the body which triggers an inflammatory pathway that results in the release of leukotrienes which cause bronchoconstriction and mucus production. Leukotrienes are considered to be one thousand times more potent than histamine and cause an asthmatic great distress.

Over a two-week period, Serge's allergens were eliminated from his diet, food preparation shifted to home-cooked meals, and the vitamin and acidophilus protocol was established. These changes resulted in dramatic improvement. The stomachaches were gone and he was sleeping through the night but still used his inhaler regularly.

We then started him on intravenous vitamins and minerals. He began with one IV every week for six weeks progressing to one IV every other week for two months and finishing with one IV every month for three months.

As of this writing, Serge is free of asthma symptoms. Since his last IV three months ago, he has not had any illnesses and has had to use his inhaler only once. He is no longer napping during the day and his stomachaches are a thing of the past.

Dr. Holk's Rx

The case study presented illustrates the naturopathic approach to heath care. The initial step in working with any patient is to determine the obstacles to healing and remove them. In this case, Serge's allergens were the most readily identifiable obstacles. The next goal is to support the natural healing of the body with nutrient-dense foods and proper supplementation. Besides oral supplementation, I highly recommend supporting asthmatics with an intravenous protocol of vitamins and minerals. With the introduction of IVs, I have seen dramatic and rapid improvement. A typical IV includes the following: magnesium, molybdenum, and B complex vitamins, with extra vitamin B_6. Vitamin B_{12} is given intramuscularly.

If you would like more information about intravenous vitamin and mineral support for your asthmatic child, have your physician contact Dr. Jonathan Wright's Tahoma Clinic at 253-854-4900 or visit the clinic's website at www.tahoma-clinic.com. Dr. Wright has authored an article in which he discusses use of vitamin B_{12} in asthma, the connection between asthma and low levels of stomach acid, and the supplementation that has proven effective. Kerry Bone, master herbalist, contributed a section on herbal protocols for the management of asthma, allergy, and inflammation. This is an invaluable resource for your physician. A copy of the article may be ordered from *www.jvwonline.com* or by calling Publishers Management Corporation at 800-528-0559.

✂ 3 ✂

Immune System Dysfunction

According to the National Center for Health Statistics (NCHS), 66 million cases of the common cold required medical attention or resulted in restricted activity in 1994 in the United States. That same year, colds also caused 20 million days lost from school. (Adams PF, Marano MA, 1995).

WHAT'S CAUSING SO MANY COLDS?

Colds are caused by more than 200 different viruses, running the gamut from mild to life-threatening. Rhinoviruses (from the Greek word *rhin*, meaning "nose") are the ones that seldom produce serious illness. They're estimated to be responsible for a third of all colds, and occur mostly in early fall, spring and summer. Another 10–15 percent of colds are caused by viruses which are responsible for more severe illness, such as Orthomyxoviruses, which contain influenza (or "flu"). The causes of 30 to 50 percent of all colds, however, remain unidentified.

WHY DOES IT SEEM THAT WE GET MORE COLDS WHEN IT *IS* COLD?

In the U.S., the autumn and winter are referred to as "cold season" for a reason – that's when most Americans get their colds. Starting in early fall, colds increase slowly and remain high until March or April, when they start to decline. This variation might correlate to the time that students return to school, as well as the increasing proportion of people staying indoors due to the colder temperatures outside. The more people are gathered indoors, the greater the likelihood of spreading (and catching!) a cold. Vitamin D, produced by sun exposure, keeps the immune system healthy. Being indoors more often in cold weather prevents absorption of this immune-boosting nutrient.

Although some people believe that a cold results from simple exposure to the outdoors, or from getting chilled or overheated, these conditions have little, if any, effect on a cold's development or intensity. Factors such as exercise, diet, enlarged tonsils or adenoids may increase susceptibility. Recent research suggests that psychological stress, allergic disorders affecting the nose and throat, and menstrual cycles may also affect whether a person will develop a cold.

HOW CAN YOU TELL WHETHER YOUR CHILD HAS A COLD OR THE FLU?

Following is a checklist from The National Institute of Allergy and Infectious Diseases:

Symptom	Cold	Flu
Fever	Rare	Usual, high (102–104 degrees F); lasts 3–4 days.
Headache	Rare	Prominent.
Fatigue, weakness	Mild	Can last up to 2–3 weeks.
Extreme Exhaustion	Rare	Early and prominent.
Complications	Sinus congestion or earache.	Bronchitis, pneumonia; can be life-threatening.
Prevention	None	Possibly annual vaccination, or antiviral drugs
Treatment	Only temporary relief of symptoms	Antiviral drugs within 24–48 hours of onset.

Source: National Institute of Allergy and Infectious Diseases, April 2001.

WHAT CAN YOU DO TO HELP *PREVENT* COLDS AND FLU FOR YOU AND YOUR CHILDREN?

1. **Wash your hands.** Spend at least twenty seconds scrubbing your hands with soap before rinsing off. (Twenty seconds is roughly the amount of time it takes to sing the "Happy Birthday" song.)

2. Get plenty of sleep. If you're tired, your immune system may be weakened.

3. Eat a healthy diet.

4. Minimize your stress level. Psychological stress does play a role in cold and flu susceptibility because it suppresses the immune system.

5. Supplement your diet with known immune system boosters. Depressed immune function may be associated with deficiencies of vitamins and minerals. Vitamin C, zinc, and selenium are particularly important.

WHAT NATURAL REMEDIES CAN BE USED TO FIGHT COLDS OR FLU?

Cold and flu viruses are everywhere. Every child, sooner or later, is exposed to a cold or flu virus, but not every child will succumb to the infection. By doing the following, you can help to strengthen and support your child's immune system when a cold or flu threatens:

- **Keep your child from eating sugary foods.** Sugar has been shown to depress the action of the immune system for up to four hours after consumption.
- **Don't fear a low-grade fever.** A low-grade fever is the body's way of creating an incompatible living environment for bacteria and viruses. When a low-grade fever is suppressed, the body has lost one of its mechanisms for disabling the invader.
- **Use antibiotics only when necessary.** Antibiotics are only effective against bacterial infections. The common cold and flu are caused by viruses, so antibiotics are useless against them. Over-prescription of antibiotics has led to antibiotic-resistant organisms which cause infections that can be devastatingly difficult to eliminate. Antibiotics also harm and/or kill the normal bacterial flora in the gut, which are so important for proper digestion, and, therefore, create an environment for gut dysfunction and all of its consequences.

- **Offer homemade chicken soup when your child is ill.** Grandma did know best! Studies have confirmed the healthful effects a bowl of homemade chicken soup can have on your child's immune system (Rennard BO, et. al., 2000). Please remember to use organic chicken, which is free of antibiotic residues. Adding lots of onions, garlic and other vegetables and cooking it with the bones will enhance its immune-boosting properties.
- **Give your child supplements.** Vitamin C, zinc in liquid (sulfate) or lozenge (gluconate – select brand with least amount of sugar added) form, and echinacea or grapefruit seed extract at the first sign of a cold or flu may reduce the severity.
- **Give your child a tepid epsom salt bath.** This type of soak can bring down a fever and reduce the muscle aches, pains, and headaches of flu.

LOW-GRADE FEVER: FRIEND OR FOE?

What is a fever? A fever is defined as a body temperature that is elevated more than two degrees Fahrenheit (98.6 degrees F. is normal). A fever can be caused by a wide variety of things, including dehydration, overexertion, an allergic or toxic reaction, or a viral or bacterial infection. Fever of an unknown origin is a condition defined as an elevated temperature lasting for a week or more without an identifiable cause. So, a fever is not a disease, but a symptom of an illness or condition. Parents are perhaps overly concerned about simple childhood fevers because of the fact that fever is a maligned and misunderstood mechanism of the body.

A fever is not necessarily a dangerous condition. It is simply a sign that the body is defending itself against an invader. Since viruses and bacteria do not survive as well in a body with an elevated temperature, a fever is actually an ally in fighting infection. It's a way that the body protects and heals itself. An elevated temperature also increases infection-fighting white blood cells, while improving their responsiveness.

A fever means a much different thing for a child than for an adult. If an adult has a high fever, this generally reflects the severity of the illness causing it. In a child, however, this is not the case. A child with pneumonia might have a fever of 100 degrees F., whereas a child with a simple cold might have a fever of 105 degrees F. If your child has a slight fever, no intervention may be necessary. Unless your child's temperature is higher than 102 degrees F., fever-reducing medication is generally not needed. Your own observation of your child's overall condition is the best indicator of its severity. Anytime a fever continues or goes above 102 degrees F. for a child, it is important to contact your child's physician. Also, if your child has a fever, **DO NOT** give him aspirin. Many fevers are caused by viral infections, and the combination of aspirin and viral illness has been linked to the development of Reye's Syndrome, a dangerous and progressively debilitating liver disease (Tierney LM, et. al., eds., 2000).

WHEN COLDS (OR OTHER INFECTIONS) BECOME CHRONIC

In chronic colds and infections, the immune system has been compromised to a point where it cannot effectively do its job and remove offending pathogens before they make the child ill. At this point, it is necessary to determine what is consistently stressing your child's immune system, and remove the stressor(s) so that the system may recover. Following are a list of questions to help you zero in on possible causes:

1. Is the overall diet healthy? Does it contain the proper balance of nutrients? A healthy diet is key to supplying the body with all of the nutrients it requires for all of the metabolic processes it undergoes each day. A healthy diet must be modified based upon your child's age and activity level (see Chapter 14 for further details).

2. Is sugar consumption high? Sugar has been shown to suppress the activity of the immune system for up to four hours after its consumption. A consistently suppressed immune system cannot properly protect your child. Further on in this chapter are details regarding the abuse of sugar.

3. Are allergies or food intolerances present? The importance of identifying triggers which may be causing a low level of chronic inflammation cannot be emphasized enough. Chronic inflammation stresses the immune system making it more difficult to respond to invaders. Chronic reaction causes inflammation in the gut. This can cause the passage of foodstuffs through inappropriate pathways (i.e., food molecules pass between cells instead of going through the cells as they should, creating an immune response to the invader that isn't recognized as "food" by the body (see Chapter 1 for more information regarding allergies and food intolerances).

4. Has a yeast overgrowth been created? This problem is widespread but frequently unsuspected because it often mimics the symptoms of sinus infections, flu, and allergies. If your child has been frequently treated with antibiotics, a yeast overgrowth may be continually suppressing your child's immune system. An elimination diet may detect this problem (see Chapter 13 for further details).

THE NOT-SO-SWEET STORY ABOUT SUGAR'S EFFECT
UPON THE IMMUNE SYSTEM

During the time of Napoleon, refined sugar was a precious commodity, desired by rich and poor alike. Since those days, the seductive properties of sugar have been immortalized in our language, forever representing something good that causes happiness; i.e. "sweetness and light," "sugar and spice and all things nice," "sweetheart," "sweet as sugar," "sweetie pie," and "sugar daddy." Our childhood memories of sugar revolve around its use as a treat or reward for good behavior or accomplishments. Our American culture is so besotted with sugar that the average citizen consumes 120-130 pounds of refined sugar each year, or a whopping 600 calories a day! Even those alert few who read the ingredients contained in their food can be misled by sugar's many aliases such as sucrose, dextrose, corn syrup, corn sugar, glucose, maltose, lactose, honey and brown sugar.

WHAT'S SO BAD ABOUT EATING REFINED SUGAR?

There are many negative effects of the consumption of refined sugar. The most devastating, however, is that consumption of refined sugar suppresses the immune system for at least four hours after consumption. This means that if one is constantly ingesting refined sugar (in any of its numerous forms), then one's immune system is constantly being suppressed. Eating whole, healthy foods allows the body to normalize its vitamin and mineral intake and strengthen its immune system.

Dr. Harold Lee Snow, who thoroughly researched and tested refined sugar, came to the following conclusions:

1. The human body does not need refined sugar. Whole natural foods supply enough carbohydrates for energy. When eating refined sugar, the body is not getting enough nutrients, so a person either has to eat more food (leading to overeating and possible obesity), or be malnourished.

2. Refined sugar is a drug or chemical, **NOT** a food. Refined sugar has been taken from a natural carbohydrate, compacted unlike any substance in nature, and treated with a myriad of chemicals during processing – such as charcoal, carbon, phosphoric acid and bleaching agents.

3. Refined sugar (like caffeine and alcohol) is habit-forming, and destroys the appetite for nourishing foods.

4. Vitamin and mineral deficiencies develop as a result of eating refined sugar. Zinc is depleted. Low levels of zinc

contribute to poor growth, acne, and depression in children and teens. Calcium and magnesium metabolism is disturbed. This affects young people the most, because teenagers, according to a recent NHANES study, consume less than 60 percent of their daily calcium requirement and even less magnesium. This lack of calcium and magnesium can contribute to decreased bone strength, leading to osteoporosis in later years. Lack of these minerals can also irritate the nervous system. This can cause muscle twitching, nervousness, irritability, fatigue, hyperactivity, and unprovoked anger.

The consumption of sugar tends to stimulate the appetite, creating a vicious cycle of overeating which results in weight gain. Obese Americans often start out as overweight children. It's important to start eliminating refined sugars from your child's diet now. This will instill good eating habits, but best of all, it will provide the necessary nutrients that your child's immune system needs to defend itself against invading pathogens. Research has shown that children who are not exposed to refined sugars until the age of two, don't tend to crave it later in life.

ANTIBIOTICS – FRIEND OR FOE?

With the production of penicillin in 1941, the "golden era" of antibiotics began. But the clinical use of antibiotics was recognized long before then. In 1877, scientists discovered that microorganisms, when threatened, secreted substances that inhibited or destroyed their "enemy." It was, and remains, as Darwin stated, "survival of the fittest." What wasn't appreciated in the early part of the century was that these microorganisms mutate or change their structure or secretions when threatened. Since these changes occur at the genetic level, this information is rapidly transferred to their offspring. This transfer of information allows the hardiest to survive against the antibiotic, therefore, making the antibiotics useless against that particular strain of bacteria.

Antibiotic resistance – the little guys are winning!

Antibiotic resistance refers to the ability of bacteria to adapt or mutate in response to a threat from their environment and, therefore, ensure their own survival. In the United States alone, there are over 150 available antibiotics, most of which are becoming useless. The Institute of Medicine, an arm of The National Academy of Sciences, states that the cost of treating antibiotic resistant infections in the United States may be as high as thirty billion dollars.

Why do bacteria become resistant?

Two factors that contribute greatly to the bacterial resistance are the overuse and misuse of antibiotics. The overuse of antibiotics occurs not only in humans but in agricultural practices as well. Many of the animal foods that we eat are given antibiotics in their feed and through injections to prevent bacterial infections and to increase the animal's productivity. When we consume these antibiotic by-products, we are weakening our own resistance to the antibiotic. Antibiotic resistant superbugs force farmers to use even more potent antibiotics.

The use of antibiotics to prevent, rather than treat, established infections is the subject of much controversy. A large percentage of the antibiotics given in the United States are used to prevent infection. There are situations where this approach is warranted, such as in organ transplants and chemotherapy. Using this same approach to prevent a secondary infection when one has a cold is not justified. The Food and Drug Association has now proposed that labels be placed on all antibiotics reminding doctors to prescribe them only when necessary.

Antibiotics are misused when they are prescribed for colds, flus or other pathologies, which are viral or fungal in nature. The Center for Disease Control (CDC) estimates that half of all antibiotics are prescribed during a visit to the doctor for colds and other viruses that cannot be treated using antibiotics. Antibiotics are only useful in treating bacterial infections and should be given for that reason and that reason alone.

The Food and Drug Administration (FDA) and Centers for Disease Control (CDC) have become so concerned about the overuse of antibiotics that they have developed an RX for physicians to use for their "antibiotic happy" patients who have viruses (see Table I) and are putting warning labels on antibiotic prescription bottles.

Name: _____ Date: ___ /___ /___

Diagnosis: ☐ Cold or Flu   ☐ Middle ear fluid (Otitis Media with Effusion, OME)
             ☐ Cough   ☐ Viral sore throat
             ☐ Other

You have been diagnosed as having illness caused by a virus. Anitbiotic treatment does not cure viral infections. If given when not needed, antibiotics can be harmful. The treatments prescribed below will help you feel better while your body's own defenses are defeating the virus.

General instructions:

☐ Increase fluids

☐ Use cool mist vaporizer or saline nasal spray to relieve congestion.

☐ Soothe throat with ice chips, or sore throat spray, lozenges for older children and adults.

Specific instructions>:

☐ Fever or aches

☐ Ear pains

Use medicines as directed by your doctor or the package instructions. Stop the medication when the symptoms get better

Follow up:
☐ If not improved in ___ days, if new sypmtoms occur or of you have other concerns, please call or return to the office for a recheck.

☐ Other _____

_____

Signed   _____

CDC

TABLE I.
Source: Centers for Disease Control

Another misuse of antibiotics occurs when a full course is not taken. It is of utmost importance to finish a course of antibiotics even if you or your child begins to feel better after only a few days. Ceasing to take all of the pills results in the quick destruction of the more susceptible bacteria but allows the less susceptible or more resistant bacteria to thrive. Taking the whole course of antibiotics helps to ensure that all of the organisms have been destroyed decreasing the probability that resistance will occur.

SUPERINFECTIONS

Superinfections are relatively common. They are secondary infections that emerge during the treatment of a primary bacterial infection. These secondary infections are not limited to bacterial infections. Many of them are fungal, e.g., *Candida Albicans*, and very difficult to treat with antiinfective agents. These infections are thought to be the result of disruption in the normal bacterial flora that inhabits the gastrointestinal, respiratory and genitourinary tracts. Because antibiotics kill the "good" bacteria as well as the "bad" bacteria, a superinfection becomes very likely. **Broad spectrum** antibiotics are the most troublesome because they have a greater adverse effect on the normal flora. An antibiotic that is specific for one organism will not cause as great a disruption in the flora.

THE IMPORTANCE OF REESTABLISHING HEALTHY FLORA DURING AND AFTER ANTIBIOTIC THERAPY

Since the "good" bacteria/healthy flora are important for proper digestion and absorption of nutrients, it is imperative that the healthy flora be replaced during or after antibiotic therapy. It is interesting to note that many of the symptoms associated with a "bad" bacterial overgrowth are also the common side effects seen with anti-biotic therapy. Supplementation of *Lactobacillus acidophilus*, the same healthy flora found in active culture yogurts, can help to offset the severity of the adverse effects and promote improved gut health. Poor gut health is now being implicated in a number of chronic conditions including asthma, allergies, anemia, chronic diarrhea, fatigue, immune system dysfunctions/chronic infections, depression and digestive disturbances (see Chapters 1 and 2 for further details).

SIDE EFFECTS OF USING ANTIBIOTICS

Table II identifies adverse reactions to antibiotics and compares them to symptoms often seen with a bacterial and/or yeast overgrowth.

HOW TO PROTECT A CHILD WHO MUST TAKE ANTIBIOTICS

- Make sure your child is taking antibiotics for a bacterial infection. A culture may have to be done to confirm this. As long as your child's illness is not life threatening, get a culture to identify the infecting organism and the antibiotic that will be most effective in killing it.

- Ask your physician to prescribe the antibiotic that is most specific for the organism identified. If at all possible, avoid broad-spectrum antibiotics, as they are more harmful to the healthy flora in the body.

- Once an antibiotic is prescribed, make sure the whole course of the prescription is taken. Do not stop in the middle of a course even if your child is feeling better. Doing so may result in result in promoting antibiotic resistant bacteria.

- Have your physician review the side effects that the drug may cause. Some antibiotics cause permanent damage, especially if taken over a long period of time. Tetracycline, for instance, can cause permanent tooth discoloration and decreased skeletal growth due to its ability to leech calcium from the body. Erythromycin can cause hearing loss.

- Don't consider antibiotic therapy for teenage acne. There are many other as effective or more effective measures for this condition. Daily use of antibiotics for acne can cause very resistant Candida infections that may take years to correct.

- **DO CALL YOUR PHYSICIAN IMMEDIATELY** if your child develops any severe side effects to an antibiotic including skin rashes, severe itching, joint swelling, shortness of breath or chest tightness, seizures, severe diarrhea, hearing loss, headaches or tremors.

- Supplement with *Lactobacillus acidophilus* in order to support and re-establish the presence of the healthy gut flora.

TABLE **II.** ADVERSE REACTIONS OF ANTIBIOTICS COMPARED TO SYMPTOMS OF BACTERIAL/YEAST OVERGROWTH

Side effects of antibiotic therapy
Abdominal discomfort
Nausea/Vomiting
Diarrhea
Allergic reactions
Skin rashes
Fever and chills
Loss of appetite
Source: Katzung BG. ed. *Basic & Clinical Pharmacology.* 6th ed., 1995.

Symptoms of bacterial/yeast overgrowth
Abdominal Cramps
Nausea
Diarrhea
Bloating and/or Flatulence (intestinal gas)
Fatty stools
Vitamin B12 malabsorption and deficiency
Weight loss
Source: Pizzorno JE, Murray MT. *Textbook of Natural Medicine,* 2nd ed., 1999.

Less common side effects of antibiotics
Liver damage
Kidney damage
Cardiovascular problems
Deafness
Bone marrow suppression
Sources: Katzung BG. ed. *Basic & Clinical Pharmacology.* 6th ed., 1995.
Jones CLA. The Antiobiotic Alternative. 2000.

Personal Case Study #3

Barbara was seven-years-old when she began experiencing painful constipation and chronic bladder infections. She had more than twenty courses of antibiotics since birth for ear and upper respiratory infections. The antibiotics that were prescribed for her bladder infections were totally ineffective. Barbara also experienced so much nausea, flatulence, fatigue, bloating, and abdominal discomfort that she had missed more than three weeks of second grade when her parents brought her to my office in December.

It was clear that Barbara had a systemic yeast imbalance. Her bladder infections were yeast, not bacterial, in nature. This was the reason for the ineffectiveness of the antibiotics. I explained to Barbara that her cravings for sugar, pretzels, bread, and soft drinks were due to her yeast problem, and that to get well, she would have to avoid them completely. She would have to eat more protein, vegetables, and healthy fats (such as avocado, nuts, and seeds) to help her get well. I also gave her lactobacillus acidophilus, grapefruit seed extract, vitamin C, zinc, and a multiple vitamin/ mineral as supplements to stimulate her immune system.

She never had another bladder infection. Her digestive symptoms improved in ten days. She also lost fifteen pounds of excess fluid within three months. After six months, Barbara could eat an occasional sugary snack and one yeast-producing food daily. She now feels in control because she knows how much she can eat of these foods without feeling the symptoms return. She also found, to her amazement, that she doesn't even miss overly processed foods, except at parties.

Dr. Holk's Rx: Grapefruit Seed Extract

This antibacterial, antiviral, antimicrobial substance, derived from organically grown grapefruit seeds, is a safe and effective compound to strengthen the immune system and to fight colds, flu, and even traveler's diarrhea. It is also excellent to treat fungal problems, such as Candida albicans and oral thrush. The drops can be used orally as a dental rinse and throat gargle. They can also be used as an ear, nasal, or vaginal rinse. The tablets are effective anytime for yeast overgrowth and as a preventive and treatment during the cold and flu season.

⫷ 4 ⫸

Attention Deficit Disorder and Other Learning and Behavior Disorders

ADHD DIAGNOSTIC CRITERIA

Although the name has changed several times since the 1970s, the health condition encompassing impulsive or inattentive behavior is now clinically referred to as Attention-Deficit/Hyperactivity Disorder or ADHD. This health problem can also affect adults, but my focus will be on children. My comments will encompass those who are only inattentive and those who are both hyperactive and inattentive.

To be diagnosed clinically with ADHD, a school-aged child needs to have exhibited at least two-thirds of the behaviors listed in Table I in one or both columns for at least six months.

TABLE I: SYMPTOMS OF AN ADHD CHILD

With Hyperactivity (Impulsive)	Without Hyperactivity (Inattentive)
Is fidgety and squirms in seat.	Has difficulty following instructions.
Leaves seat when shouldn't.	Has difficulty paying attention to tasks and/or play activities.
Runs or climbs inappropriately.	
Talks excessively, often inappropriately.	Loses things necessary for tasks and activities at school and at home.
Has difficulty playing quietly.	Doesn't listen.
Is always on the go.	Fails to give close attention to details.
Blurts our answers without raising hand.	Is disorganized.
Has trouble awaiting a turn.	Has trouble with tasks requiring long-term mental effort.
Interrupts or intrudes upon others.	Is forgetful in daily activities.
	Is easily distracted.

Adapted from *Hyperactivity and Attention Disorders in Children*. The Health Information Network, 1995 and The American Psychiatric Association, *Diagnostic and Statistical Manual of Mental Disorder*, 1995.

51

ADHD ON THE RISE

ADHD is one of the fastest growing childhood disorders in the United States; it is also a problem virtually unheard of in many other countries. By the year 2000, about 8 million children, an astounding 20 percent of the entire school age population, were diagnosed with this disorder and treated with stimulants. At least 13 million adults have also been diagnosed with this disorder "du jour" (U.S. Drug Enforcement Agency (DEA), National Institutes of Health, Washington D.C.). Many government experts, including those at DEA and the National Institute of Mental Health (NIMH) are concerned that ADHD is being overdiagnosed with patients being overmedicated. Gene Haislip, a former deputy assistant administrator at DEA, asked in his December 1996 DEA address, *Why are we rushing to feed stimulants (such as methylphenidate in the form of Ritalin®) to children?* The United States uses five times more Ritalin® than the rest of the world combined.

The National Institutes of Health (NIH) is now funding a multi-million dollar study of ADHD children and the effects of Ritalin®. It is shocking to realize that studies are being performed **after** medicating children instead of before to prove safety and efficacy.

Although I have often seen an ADHD label made by a teacher to then be diagnosed by the child's pediatrician, parents should accept the ADHD diagnosis only if a team of professionals (i.e., psychologists, psychiatrists, and social workers specializing in this disorder) has agreed upon the diagnosis. The pediatrician's, internists', or general practitioner's role should be only to rule out other medical conditions that could account for the symptoms. For instance, many overdiagnosed children were suffering from debilitating allergies, headaches, or profound hearing loss when diagnosed with ADHD. After their physical problem was corrected, the ADHD behavior disappeared.

To date, brain imaging techniques have provided clues as to the cause of ADHD, but there are no definitive laboratory tests to identify markers. A Boston company says they have identified a clear-cut chemical abnormality in ADHD children and have developed a diagnostic agent, dubbed Altropane. It is now in clinical trials. If this diagnostic test proves effective, ADHD will probably be diagnosed more scientifically, and less subjectively in the future.

WHY IS THERE A SURGE IN HYPERACTIVITY?

Most experts feel that the following factors play a role in hyperactivity:

1. **Emotional/ Relationship Issues**
   - Lack of physical touching, expressions of caring and love
   - Parents not sharing activities and interests with children
   - Parents and teachers not helping children to channel their energy in positive ways
   - Parents and teachers not allowing enough calming, quiet activities (i.e., listening to soft music, massage, reading books)

2. **Diet**
   - Refined sugar products (soft drinks, candy, cookies, cakes, pastries, honey, dried fruits, fruit juice) and overabundance of simple carbohydrates, especially from sweetened snacks. A sugar "challenge" administered with a high carbohydrate breakfast (i.e. sugared cereal, milk and orange juice) has been proven to reduce the attention span of normal and hyperactive children alike. (Conners, C.K., 1989).
   - Overly processed foods containing harmful food additives. A diet of "dead" foods produces mineral imbalances, essential fatty acids deficiencies, osteopathic problems, and neurological disorganization, all of which can affect learning and behavior.

- Food reactors (the most common are pasteurized dairy products, eggs, glutenous grains, yeast, corn, and salicylates)
- Impaired glucose metabolism. Scientists at the National Institutes of Mental Health feel that impaired glucose metabolism may be a major problem contributing to ADHD. It is now known that American children eat too many simple carbohydrates and too many nutrient-poor foods (that lack magnesium and zinc, both essential for carbohydrate metabolism).

3. **Environmental Factors**
   - Exposure to toxic substances. The U.S. Congress and The Office of Technology Assessment wrote *Neurotoxicity: Identifying and Controlling Poisons of the Nervous System* (U.S. Govt. Printing Office) in 1990. Among other concerns, they mentioned *that toxic substances can contribute to neuropsychiatric disorders. The National Academy of Sciences recently reported (in 1990) that 12 percent of the 63 million children under the age of 18 in the U.S. suffer from one or more mental disorders and it identified exposure to toxic substances before or after birth as one of the several risk factors* (Neurotoxicity, page 8). Why have the Environmental Protection Agency and the Food and Drug Administration virtually ignored governmental concerns and their plea for more scientific studies to assess this matter?
   - Heavy metal contamination (including lead from house paint or mercury from many sources, including vaccines and amalgam dental fillings)
   - Artificial lighting (in schools, a study showed a major improvement in hyperactivity when fluorescent lights were removed from classrooms)
   - Strong electromagnetic fields
   - Noise pollution (including digital sound from computers, video games, and CD players)

For most children, a two-week elimination diet (see Chapter 13 for details) that avoids all common food toxins and allergens while providing balance of protein, carbohydrates, and fats, can tell parents definitively whether diet can be a causative factor. Ninety-five percent of all the ADHD children I have worked with, including my own daughter, have shown a remarkable improvement during the second week of this nutritional elimination plan.

WHY DON'T MORE PARENTS TRY AN ELIMINATION DIET?

To rule out diet as a major cause of ADHD, it seems so simple to focus on a healthy diet that avoids food reactors. But, sadly, most parents don't know that diet is important because the largest organization of children and adults with Attention Deficit Disorder, CHADD, ridicules dietary factors. The fact that their funding comes primarily from stimulant drug companies should make families suspicious. In addition, schools and medical practitioners will often tell parents that diets have nothing to do with ADHD and ridicule parents who refuse to medicate. I have also seen parents who aren't willing to make the necessary changes after the dietary problems are identified. They would rather use a quick fix to solve the problem. Unfortunately, medication alone has never solved the underlying imbalance, it only masks the imbalance until it resurfaces as an emotional disorder, alcoholism, obesity, and/or drug dependency later in life.

RITALIN® ROBOTS

Prescriptions of Ritalin® given to children with ADHD jumped 700 percent this decade and the United States uses 90 percent of the worldwide Ritalin® supply, according to the National Institutes of Health (NIH). Although more than 25 possible reactions to Ritalin® are listed in The *Physician's Desk Reference*, most prescribing physicians downplay them. Reduced appetite, weight loss, slowed growth, nausea, headaches, insomnia, and suicidal behavior when going on and off the medication (i.e., weekends and school holidays) are common reactions that warrant serious medical discussion.

Dr. Lawrence Diller, the author of *Running on Ritalin, A Physician Reflects on Children, Society, and Performance* (September, 1998) pointed out the drug industry's hand in creating this disorder to promote Ritalin® sales. Class action suits filed in New Jersey and California allege a conspiracy between the pharmaceutical industry, physicians, and the leading ADHD self-help group, CHADD, to unnecessarily push this medication to children. In fact, the manufacturer of Ritalin® admitted in 1995 that CHADD received one million dollars from them for their projects. In a statement made by Peter Breggin, M.D., in a lawsuit against Ritalin® he said, *Novartis (the manufacturer of Ritalin®) has unethically used its money to finance a group that would directly promote additive drugs (San Diego Union Tribune,* March 5, 2001). Practically every researcher of ADHD now accepts drug company money, as do self-help groups, with the exception of The Feingold Association.

Adderall®, the "new amphetamine on the block," has now surpassed Ritalin® as the ADHD amphetamine of choice. The effects are essentially the same as Ritalin®, differing mainly in their duration of action, according to the 1992 issue of *Psychiatric Clinic of North America.*

Before you, as parents, are pressured to give your child amphetamines (i.e., Ritalin®, Dexedrine®, Adderal®, Desoxyn®, Cylert®, Gradument®) to enhance school performance, keep in mind that:

- Amphetamines don't correct biochemical imbalances – they cause them.
- Amphetamines can cause gross abnormalities in brain function.
- Labeling children with ADHD and treating them with amphetamines can keep them out of the Armed Services and limit future careers, besides stigmatizing them for life.

- Amphetamines can cause the same negative effects as the amphetamine, cocaine, including behavior disorders, growth suppression, neurological tics, agitation, addiction, and psychosis. In fact, there has been some evidence of a higher cocaine usage among teens and adults who were on amphetamines for ADHD.

Adapted from Peter Breggin, M.D.'s *Talking Back to Ritalin®: What Doctor's Aren't Telling You About Stimulants for Children*. Common Courage Press, 1998.

It is also important for parents to realize that the safety and efficacy of long-term use of stimulants for children have never been tested (*Physician's Desk Reference*, 2000). Parents who are pressured into using behavior-modifying drugs for their child by their pediatrician should find a new pediatrician who embraces integrative methods, including dietary improvements. At the same time, they should copy the research references from this chapter connecting nutrition to learning and behavior and present it to any close-minded health practitioners they encounter. Parents who are forced to use drugs for their child by their child's school should find another school or form of education (i.e., private school or home schooling).

NUTRITION: THE BEST MEDICINE

The esteemed Center for Science in the Public Interest, a nonprofit health-advocacy organization, made a plea in their 1999 *Diet, ADHD, and Behavior* publication stating that *Government, private agencies, and health practitioners concerned about children with ADHD and other behavioral problems, should acknowledge the potential for diet to affect behavior and should advise parents to consider modifying their child's diet as a first means of treatment.* The Feingold Association of America (FAUS) reiterates this message, by encouraging and assisting parents to try a salicylate-free diet (see Chapter 13 for further details). For any family who has witnessed improvement with a salicylate-free diet, I urge you to become a member of FAUS (703-768-3287). FAUS can help make your food plan easy to follow and provide a great deal of support to families just starting their dietary changes.

According to William Walsh, Ph.D. (senior research scientist of the Health Resource Institute and the Pfeiffer Treatment Center in Naperville, Illinois), many psychiatrists look at nutritional therapies and behavior disorders with scorn. Dr. Walsh's question for them is – where do neurotransmitters come from? They can only come from nutrients such as amino acids, vitamins, and minerals. If the brain receives the improper amounts of these building blocks, we can see serious problems with neurotransmitters, which will affect serotonin, dopamine, norepinephrine, and other brain chemicals (Walsh, *NOHA News*, 2000).

I have had fabulous success instituting dietary changes with families after addressing food sensitivity or allergies. I always encourage the whole family to make changes together so that the household presents a united front. I can't tell you how many times chronic health conditions disappear among other family members when positive dietary changes are made for the whole family.

Following are the steps I usually recommend for children who have behavioral and learning issues:

- **Follow a two-week elimination diet to rule out food sensitivities/allergies** (see Chapter 13 for details). This is best done under the direction of a knowledgeable health professional. After we discover the problem(s), we address what we can through diet, and refer to specialists if further testing is warranted. In my experience, salicylate sensitivity with one or more food allergies and/or impaired glucose metabolism is present in about 50 percent of my cases. Yeast overgrowth (if the child has been on repeated courses of antibiotics) with environmental allergies usually manifests as 30 percent of my cases. About 10 percent of the children I see experience all of these reactions. Another 10 percent have nutritional deficiencies from living on protein poor "dead foods." I have never worked with an ADHD child who had none of these conditions, even when the parents were certain that the child had no nutritional issues.

- **Plan a healthy diet for your child, free of any known triggers.** It is usually best if "house cleaning" is performed to remove all trigger items. If other family members can tolerate the child's trigger foods, it is usually best to eat them out and away from the child.

- **Balance proteins, carbohydrates, and fats for your child.** Train your child to always eat a protein and/or fat when eating a carbohydrate for blood sugar balance. ADHD children usually crave carbohydrates and hate proteins. It may take some "retraining," but the balance issue will become second nature when your child knows it is a new rule. The added benefits are a child with more **positive** energy, more emotional control, and optimum weight.

- **Avoid fruit juice.** Juices contain too much natural sugar and most contain salicylates. Even the American Pediatric Association recommends no juice for babies younger than six months, no more than six ounces of juice for children six and younger, and eight to twelve ounces maximum for children aged seven to eighteen. A much better idea is to enlist your child in helping you make fruit smoothies. These are a balance of protein, carbohydrate, and fat, and are especially recommended as a breakfast substitute or snack when your child doesn't feel very hungry. The following salicylate-free recipes have always been a big hit in our household.

Power Pina Colada
>   1 cup coconut milk (a "brain food")
>   1 cup plain organic yogurt or enriched plain soymilk
>   1 large very ripe banana, sliced
>   ½ cup crushed pineapple with juice
>   15–20 grams whey, soy, or rice protein powder
>   Crushed ice, to taste

Blend all in blender or food processor. Serve immediately or freeze for power popsicles.

Chocolate Banana Freeze
>   1 cup chocolate enriched soymilk, organic full fat plain yogurt,
>   or rice milk with 1 tsp. cocoa powder and 1 tsp. pure maple syrup
>   ½ very ripe banana, sliced
>   15–20 grams whey, soy, or rice protein powder
>   Water or ice chips, to taste

Blend all in blender or food processor. Serve immediately or freeze in 6–8 oz. paper cups.

For other drink choices, filtered mineral water (sparkling or plain) is the best recommendation. Eight to sixteen ounces of enriched and calcium-fortified soy milk, oat milk, almond milk, and rice milk are other daily drink options.

Avoid artificial colors, chemicals, preservatives, monosodium glutamate, and aspartame for the whole family. These may not only cause serious reactions, but can alter brain chemistry.

Follow a non-allergenic vitamin/mineral supplement regimen. The following nutrients should be included:

> **B Vitamins:** The whole complex is necessary, but I particularly recommend between 10-50 mg. of B_6, based on the child's height, weight, and allergy profile. Two excellent double-blind studies comparing B vitamins to Ritalin® found the B vitamins were more effective, safer, and cheaper. It is important for children to take magnesium with B-vitamins for proper absorption.

> **Magnesium:** 75 percent of all people living in the United States are magnesium deficient. Clinicians

in Europe have also found lower than normal levels of magnesium in the red blood cells for most people with ADHD. Magnesium is "nature's valium." It calms, reduces irritability, stops muscle tension and spasms, promotes restful sleep, and increases exercise tolerance. It is also an essential partner to B-6, and reduces allergic reactions.

I usually recommend between 100–400 mg. daily in a highly absorbable form, such as glycinate. If a child cannot tolerate enough orally, I recommend Epsom Salt Baths (Magnesium Sulfate) nightly. We use 2–4 cups in warm water for a 15 minute soak.

Essential Fatty Acids (EFAs): Children who have dry skin and hair, brittle nails, and excessive thirst without excessive urination are usually low in EFAs. Fish and flax oils are my two favorite recommendations in the form of Cod Liver Oil (liquid or capsules) and Flax Oil (liquid or capsules). Some children require all of the EFAs (Omega 3, 6 and 9). It is best to consult a licensed health professional to assist your child with EFAs.

DHA (Docosahexaenoic acid): DHA is a very important essential fatty acid for optimum cognitive function. In Europe, all baby formulas contain DHA because it is known to raise I.Q. levels by as much as twelve points. There is now grass roots pressure to incorporate DHA into all baby formulas in the United States. The most common source is high oleic safflower or sunflower oil. In my practice, I usually recommend adding one of these oils to rice or soymilk for children over the age of twelve months. I also recommend cold water fatty fish such as salmon, sardines, tuna, or mackerel as a good source of DHA and EFAs. If a child will not consume these food sources regularly, I usually recommend a DHA supplement called Neuromins.

DMAE: Although I usually don't recommend this supplement, I approve of its use under doctor's orders. Most doctors recommend this supplement to make choline (found in B-vitamin supplements, egg yolks, and soy lecithin), a neurotransmitter used for memory and thinking. To improve learning and behavior, a dose of 600-1200 mg. daily is usually recommended.

Check iron status: Low iron is the most common cause of poor concentration and distractibility among American children. A Complete Blood Count (CBC) can easily detect iron deficiency anemia. If low, short-term iron (the ferrous form) supplement use, while changing your child's diet, may be necessary. Low iron and low ferritin (protein-bound iron) are the major causes of poor concentration but very seldom detected by the medical profession. I witnessed a bizarre case in which a psychotherapist mother and client of mine told that me her three-year-old daughter had been diagnosed with psychotic behavior and was given a prescription for Prozac®. The child was noted to be gnawing on wooden objects (window sills, legs of chairs, etc.). I asked the mother what the CBC showed because it sounded like Pica, a disorder manifesting in eating non-food items. Pica is often caused by mineral deficiencies. The mother asked, "What CBC?" The psychiatrist had not ordered one. When I insisted, her pediatrician ordered a CBC to find, to her dismay, that the child suffered from acute protein and iron deficiency anemia. Once corrected, the "wood gnawing psychosis" stopped.

Check zinc status: Zinc is often low in ADHD children. Zinc is critical for concentration. Low zinc can easily be detected with a taste test (if zinc is low, the liquid zinc tastes like water). Metagenics Zinc Tally, Ethical Nutrients Zinc Status and Thorne Research Liquid Zinc are available sources to test your child's zinc level. In young children (under the age of seven), we continue using the liquid zinc daily while providing zinc-rich foods (fish and sunflower seeds, in particular). When the child notices a bitter taste, we discontinue supplemental use while checking it periodically. With older children, we usually supplement with 10–20 mg. daily in pill or lozenge form.

Please note: If iron and zinc supplements are taken together, they may compete for absorption. I always recommend taking supplemental iron several hours away from all other minerals.

Rule out heavy metal contamination: Blood tests can rule out lead and mercury toxicity. If toxicity levels are high, chelation therapy can remove lead, although it cannot reverse the damage. Other natural therapies are on the horizon for gradually reversing the damage.

CAN A HEALTHY NUTRITIONAL PROGRAM HELP CHILDREN WHO AREN'T LEARNING OR BEHAVIORALLY CHALLENGED?

Because most families follow my recommendations to lend support to their "challenged child," we usually see remarkable improvements in grades, energy, athletic ability, and self-esteem among the other children in the family. Following the regimen provides sharing, support, and caring that all humans need. It also shows that every child is unique and may have different needs that they can control. Some family members stopped having stomachaches, others lost weight, and others stopped having chronic colds. Controlling even one aspect of one's life can provide power and greater self-esteem. We very seldom see children who have had to watch their food intake at an early age turning to alcohol and drugs as teens because they are already "high on life."

What would have happened if health professionals had forced drugs upon Thomas Alva Edison or Martin Luther King, both of whom could have been diagnosed with ADHD if living today? A national slogan of "Hugs, not Drugs" might stand up to the billion-dollar drug business that pushes legal drugs upon our children instead of exploring natural alternatives. Let's give our kids a chance and show our love and support by working hard to provide them with nutrient-dense contaminant-free foods. Our children's new motto should be: *If you love me, don't feed me junk* (Adapted from John Robbin's *Reclaiming Our Health: Exploring the Medical Myth and Embracing the Source of True Healing.* H.J. Kramer, Inc., 1996).

Personal Case Study #4

Stephen was a six-year-old terror when his mother first brought him in. He was impossible in school. He had even threatened a girl with a kitchen knife he had brought on the bus when he as five-years-old. He dumped water out of our waiting room cooler, knocked down and confiscated two sets of business cards, and came into my office kicking and screaming. Needless to say, it was a trying visit, but I knew attempting to reason with him while he was in a "fight or flight" mode was senseless. He had eaten artificially flavored chewy candy fifteen minutes before our appointment. After sending him home with his babysitter, I explained the supplement regimen and Elimination Diet to his mother, who was desperate to try anything except medication.

Three weeks later, Stephen came into my office again. Very bright and inquisitive, he was rational, focused, and attentive during this visit. I actually enjoyed his company. The entire family was impressed with his behavior and learning improvements, but he was more pleased that his itching (he described it as "bugs crawling all over under my skin") and headaches were gone. We discovered salicylates, yeast, wheat, and cow's milk products as triggers, each manifesting in different ways. It was clearly the salicylates, however, that caused the out-of-control, violent behavior. Even his school has admitted that his learning and behavioral improvements are nothing short of remarkable. He usually is very compliant with his diet because he hates being "bad."

Dr. Holk's Natural Rx

Biofeedback is a therapeutic modality that uses electronic instruments to measure and process physiological responses that are usually outside of conscious awareness and control. Some of the processes when brought to conscious awareness, through the use of auditory or visual feedback, can be influenced by voluntary control. It's this voluntary control over mental and physiological processes that makes biofeedback an important modality in many disorders.

In a typical biofeedback session, sensors from electronic or electromechanical instruments (electromyography (EMG) and peripheral skin temperature are the principle modalities used today) are attached to the surface of the skin at various locations on the body, usually the fingers, shoulders, head and back. Electrical impulses from these locations are recorded and reflected on a computer monitor in the form of graphs or other visual displays. The client may also receive auditory feedback, which reflects increases or decreases in body system activity. The auditory feedback is usually in the form of musical tones. The purpose of measuring these impulses is to recognize physiological responses and learn to alter them. Clients can learn to control their heart rate, breathing, body temperature, blood flow, and fluid regulation.

EEG, another type of biofeedback, monitors brain waves. Brain wave measurements are recorded through silver discs commonly placed at four locations on the scalp. These measurements reflect different mental states such as attention and concentration. This form of biofeedback is helpful in treating ADD and ADHD, anxiety disorders, and other problems relating to behavior.

Current research shows biofeedback to be useful in reducing symptoms of migraine headaches (Sargent, Green and Walters, 1972), tension headaches (Budzynski and Stoyva, 1969, 1970), test anxiety (Garrett and Silver, 1972), neck and shoulder pain, Raynaud's syndrome

(Surwit, 1973), attention deficit and hyperactivity disorders, seizure activity (Sterman, 1973) stomach acidity (Gorman and Kamiya, 1972), asthma (Benson, Shapiro, Tursky, and Schwartz, 1971), and anxiety disorders.

Biofeedback is recognized among health practitioners as an effective, safe and powerful therapeutic tool that teaches patients to self-regulate certain body functions thereby reducing unwanted side effects of certain disorders.

For more information about biofeedback, contact:

Association for Applied Psychophysiology and Biofeedback at *http://www.aapb.org/public/articles/details.cfm?id=7*

Bio Research Institute at *http://www.7hz.com/sho.html*

Leonard Holmes, Ph.D.; Mental Health Resources at *http://mentalhealth.about.com/library/weekly/aa092099.htm*

To locate a certified biofeedback practitioner in your area, contact the Biofeedback Certification Institute of America (*http://www.bcia.org/generalinfo_findpractitioner.cfm*) When contacting a new practitioner, they suggest asking the following questions to insure selecting the best practitioner for your child's health needs:

- Does the professional have experience and success treating your child's symptoms/disorder?
- How many children has the practitioner successfully treated? How many of those children had the same problem(s) your child has?
- What is the length and cost of the proposed treatment?
- How long has the practitioner been doing biofeedback?
- What are the practitioner's other professional competencies?
- What other disorders does the practitioner specialize in treating?
- Are professional references available?

⁓℃ 5 ℈⁓

Autism Spectrum Disorders

THE AUTISM EPIDEMIC

In the last several years, there has been a dramatic increase in the number of cases of autism. Bernard Rimland, founder and director of the Autism Research Institute and founder of the Autism Society of America, states that autism has been on the rise since the late 1980's. Cases of autism, once considered rare and having an occurrence rate of one in 1500, continue to rise. Current estimates show that one in 500 children have autism, with recent studies in California and New Jersey showing evidence of as many as one in 150 may suffer from Autism Spectrum Disorders (Rimland B, 2000). The U.S. Department of Education reports the number of autistic students from 1994 to 1999 rose 136 percent (Beaupre B, 2000). Most alarming, are the emerging reports of the onset of autistic symptoms after the administration of multiple vaccines, most notably, the measles, mumps and rubella (MMR) vaccination.

To address this issue, the National Immunization Program (NIP), an arm of the Center for Disease Control and Prevention (CDC), has begun to support new research in this area. In 1997, the National Institutes of Health began a five year international collaborative network to study the neurobiology and genetics of autism. The National Institute of Child Health and Human Development (NICHD) and the National Institute on Deafness and Other Communicative Disorders (NIDCD) are leading the effort. At present there is no available scientific data that supports a correlation between the MMR vaccine and autism (Vastag B, 2001; Marshall H, 2001; Marwick C, 2001; Ashraf H, 2001) except for the well publicized work of Dr. Andrew Wakefield of the United Kingdom (Wakefield AJ, 1999). Without scientific research to support the autism/vaccination theory, our government agencies are slow to embrace any change in the current immunization recommendations set by the NIP. Yet, hundreds of letters from parents are sent to government agencies yearly describing the dramatic health changes that occurred in their child after receiving multiple vaccinations. Many of these parents have joined a growing movement of local and international health care practitioners and researchers in documenting anecdotal evidence. Results of this international effort are promising.

WHAT IS AUTISM?

The term autism refers to a developmental disability that includes a variety of behavior patterns with differing degrees of severity. Because the behavior patterns can be varied and the degree of severity can range from very mild to quite severe, the term *autism spectrum disorders* (*ASD*) is now being used to encompass both the classical form of autism (as defined in the *Diagnostic and Statistical Manual of Mental Disorders*, Fourth Edition) as well as the other related disabilities that share many of autism's defining characteristics.

Within the autism spectrum, autism or autistic disorder is the most severe. Infantile autism usually manifests within the first year of life and not later than 30 months and is more prevalent in boys than girls. Communication in autistic children may be completely nonverbal. Spoken language, if present, may be idiosyncratic and echolalic (echoing of other's words). Language, if developed, is used for self-stimulation ("stimming") rather than for communication. These children may appear deaf because of their unresponsiveness to external stimuli. Frequently, they show signs of mental retardation, although all children with autism are not necessarily mentally retarded (Schwartz MW, et. al., 1997).

TABLE I. CLASSIFICATIONS OF AUTISTIC SPECTRUM DISORDERS	
Less severe	ADD
	ADHD
	Dyslexia
	Asperger's
	Hyperlexia
	PDD
Most severe	Autism or Autistic Disorder
Source: Lemer, Mothering, 2000.	

On the other end of the spectrum are children who are able to function relatively well and show only mild impairment in communication and/or social exchange. These children, who are considered to be high functioning autistics, may have average or above average I.Q.s, and some even display superior (vocabulary) skills. Table I lists the different disorders that fall under the autistic spectrum disorder classification, based on the severity of symptoms.

THE POSSIBLE CAUSES OF AUTISTIC SPECTRUM DISORDERS

There are many plausible theories as to the cause of autism. Researchers have learned that autistic children exhibit symptoms involving many systems of the body. As varied as these symptoms can be, children within the autistic spectrum share one very important commonality-they have had many health issues early in life, including difficult births, mothers with health issues during pregnancy, recurrent ear infections with multiple antibiotic use, digestive problems and other conditions which may contribute to an overall cumulative negative affect. "Total Load Theory" refers to the cumulative effect of individual assaults of each health problem on the body as a whole (Rimland B, *Mothering*, 2000). These children may be in a weakened state at the time of receiving their first vaccinations with immature or underdeveloped immune, digestive and detoxification systems. This theory suggests that vaccinations may present as the "overload" to their system where their bodies cannot appropriately manage the added assault and damage ensues. Listed below are **risk factors** that may contribute to autistic spectrum disorders:

- Traumatic birth
- Fibromyalgia, chronic fatigue or low thyroid function in the mother
- History of an extended immunization reaction
- Sudden decline in function between 15 and 30 months
- Chronic, unexplained fevers
- Allergies in the family
- Dark circles under the eyes (allergic shiners)
- Respiratory problems, including asthma and bronchitis
- Digestive problems, including constipation, chronic diarrhea, or reflux
- Skin problems, including eczema and poor color
- Recurrent ear, sinus or strep infections
- Agitated sleep
- Yeast infections, such as thrush
- Wild swings in mood and function
- Red ears or apple cheeks
- Craving for apple juice
- Sensitivity to dyes, chemicals, perfumes or medications
- Self-injury or violent behavior
- Regressive behavior after eating food with additives

Genetics may also play a role in predisposing a child to autism. Research funded by the National Institutes of Health has identified a gene which may contribute to the development autism. The gene, identified as HOXA1, is important in early brain development and may account for some types of autism (Ingram JL, et. al., 2000).

Researchers of the DAN! (Defeat Autism Now!) Subcommittee on Mercury and Autism are convinced that toxic **heavy metals** play an important role in the development of at least some autism related symptoms. Mercury, cadmium, lead, aluminum, tin and antimony have been found at excessively high levels in autistic children. Mercury toxicity has received much public attention because of its use as a preservative (thimerosal) in vaccines (see Chapter 6 for further details). Mercury is especially dangerous at high levels because it prevents zinc from assisting in the formation of myelin basic protein (MBP). This protein is crucial for proper nerve insulation and conduction. Mercury also triggers the formation of autoantibodies that damage brain tissue (Bradstreet J, et. al., 2000). According to V.K. Singh, Ph.D., who testified at a recent Congressional hearing, approximately 80 percent of the children with autism have autoantibodies to MBP and/or Neuronal Filament Proteins (Bradstreet J, et. al., 2000; Singh VK, 1993) With repeated exposure to the ravages of mercury, children become more susceptible to other heavy metal damage as well. Mercury, found in vaccinations, amalgams, fish and other food sources, pose a direct threat to children. Consider also the prenatal exposure to maternal mercury. Data on prenatal exposure to toxins from the study of two metals, lead and mercury, have shown deleterious affects (Needleman HL, 1995).

In June of 1999, the American Academy of Pediatrics and the U.S. Public Health Service acknowledged that mercury exposure from vaccines given in the first six months of life exceeded maximum acceptable levels established by federal guidelines and called for a **phasing out** of all thimerosal-containing vaccines in the U.S. Although this is a step in the right direction, mercury-laden vaccines are still the norm in many other parts of the world, especially in developing countries. Mercury should be removed from vaccines worldwide **immediately**. Our children's health depends on it.

Vaccinations as a risk factor for autism can no longer be denied. Dan Burton, Chairman of the Government Reform Committee of the U.S. House of Representatives shared his own personal experience with autism during an April 6, 2000, presentation on *Autism: Present Challenges, Future Need – Why the Increased Rates?*. Commenting on the numerous letters he received from parents whose children became autistic after receiving multiple vaccinations, he said, *I don't have to read a letter to experience the heartbreak. I see it in my own family. My grandson, Christian, was born healthy. He was beautiful and tall. We were already planning his NBA career. He was outgoing and talkative. He enjoyed company and going places. Then, his mother took him for his routine immunizations and all of that changed. He was given what so many children were given, DtaP, OPV, Haemophilus, Hepatitis B and MMR all at one office visit. That night Christian had a slight fever and he slept for long periods of time. When he was awake he would scream a horrible high-pitched scream. He began dragging his head on the furniture and banging it repeatedly. Over the week-and-a-half after the vaccinations, Christian would stare into space and act like he was deaf. He would hit himself and others, which was something he had never done. He would shake his head from side to side as fast as he could. He lost his language* (Burton D, 2000).

The current NIP schedule for vaccinations may be too aggressive for some children and may need modifying to accommodate this select group. Some children should not be given certain vaccines, such as pertussis and combined MMR (see Chapter 6 on vaccinations for more information).

Many children with autism have poor **fatty acid metabolism**. Essential fatty acids play an important role in proper brain function. An imbalance of fatty acids in the brain can lead to improper cell communication. In addition, fatty acids help form local acting hormones called eicosanoids which help the brain with cell to cell communication. They also play a role in sleep regulation and have an effect on sedative mechanisms in the brain.

Doctors, including Dr. A. J. Richardson of the Laboratory of Physiology at Oxford University, have recognized some correlation between autistic disorders, dyslexia, dyspraxia and ADHD. Dr. Richardson suggests that fatty acid abnormalities plays an important role in neurodevelopmental disorders like ADHD and autism. Many learning disorders are now being linked to fatty acid abnormalities possibly arising from the lack of proper dietary intake and metabolic dysfunction from heavy metal exposure (Richardson AJ, Ross MA, 2000).

Children with autistic spectrum disorder tend to have **chronic digestive problems**. The symptoms of digestive disturbance often appear with emotional and behavioral changes at the onset of autism. The gastrointestinal tract plays a very important role in the health of the immune and nervous systems. It is the first line of defense against unfriendly microbes. Any compromise in its integrity can cause deleterious effects.

The consumption of compatible foods to promote optimal digestion is the first step in helping the gut to heal. Proper absorption of broken down food particles into tissues of the GI tract is dependent upon proper pH levels, an intact tissue lining and a balanced microflora within the gut. When any of these are compromised, poor digestion, malabsorption and poor assimilation occur. The result is "leaky gut," which manifests as flatulence, bloating, irregular bowel movements, food sensitivities, yeast overgrowth, vitamin and mineral deficiencies and more. Children with autistic spectrum disorders can have one or all of these imbalances.

Children with autistic spectrum disorders exhibit many **nutritional deficiencies**. Calcium, magnesium, iron, vitamin B_1, vitamin B_6, vitamin B_{12}, glutathione and antioxidant deficiencies have all been implicated (Hoffman, RL, 1996). Poor protein intake, poor fat metabolism (too many hydrogenated fats with too few essential fatty acids), and excess carbohydrate consumption also play a role in poor nutritional status.

WHAT DIETARY SUGGESTIONS CAN IMPROVE CHILDREN WITH AUTISM?

Diet has become the main focus of treatment of most progressive doctors treating the Autistic Spectrum Disorders. Autistic children do especially well on gluten-free (off wheat and most grains), casein-free (off dairy products) diets. Betsy Prohaska, private dietary consultant, has written a book with accompanying videotape, giving tips on how to implement a gluten/casein free diet. (847-854-6601; prohaska@mc.net). She recommends increasing the intake of protein, organic meats, vegetables, healthy fats, beans, seeds, nuts and filtered water. In addition to a gluten/casein free diet, foods should be free of yeast, mold, processed sugar, artificial colors, flavors and additives. Foods with naturally occurring salicylates like apple juice should also be avoided (Lemer PS, 2000). The Feingold Association of the United States (FAUS) provides information on diets without artificial colors, flavors or preservatives (to contact FAUS: 800-321-FAUS; www.feingold.org).

Because autistic children have poor absorption, impaired immune systems, impaired ability to detoxify environmental toxins and possible inherited nutrient deficiencies, nutritional supplementation has been shown to be helpful (Lemer PS, 2000). B-vitamins, magnesium, digestive enzymes, probiotics, vitamin C, and zinc are especially important and prescribed by most progressive health professionals working with autistic children.

Secretin is a digestive aid that may be helpful for autistic children. NBC Dateline's film segment about Parker Beck, a three-year-old boy suffering from autism and chronic digestive problems, stimulated new research to better understand how **secretin**, an intestinal hormone which helps regulate stomach acid/base balance, can improve brain function. Parker's speech and sociability skills were restored when he was treated with secretin. Some children have shown great success with this substance; others have not. If well monitored by a knowledgeable physician, it is usually worth trying.

WHERE DO WE GO FROM HERE?

With so much national and international research currently underway, it is important to stay updated to fully understand the best method of treatment for the Autism Spectrum Disorders. It is promising to see hundreds of researchers and medical doctors working to find causes and cures. While not yet scientifically validated, the vaccination theory/controversy needs further investigation to determine why so many new cases of autism seem to be associated with the administration of vaccinations. Children in the autistic spectrum can have immunological, dermatological, digestive, sensory, neurological, respiratory, cognitive, psychological and/or developmental anomalies. These symptoms vary with each case of autism. Given the complexity of autism spectrum disorders, proper diagnosis and individualized treatment plans designed to address the unique symptoms of each autistic case are crucial.

Personal Case Study #5

Phillip was two and a half years old when his devastated mother reported that he had just been diagnosed with autism. He had manifested digestive problems and chronic ear infections since he had been switched from breast-feeding to milk formula at six-months of age, but he had been developing normally. The day after his MMR injection, he stopped interacting with his parents and other children. In addition, his digestive problems escalated into chronic diarrhea. Although Phillip's mother was aware, as a nurse, that there were medications to stop his diarrhea, she wanted to find its cause.

An elimination diet revealed that his most serious physical reaction was to all cow's milk products except butter. In addition, avoidance of yeasty foods, sugar, and all grains except rice, stopped the diarrhea and reduced Phillip's autistic symptoms markedly. In fact, he had completely stopped his "stimming" behavior until we introduced a whole-wheat cracker in my office.

Phillip is one of my few success stories for children with autism. Between megadoses of nutrients; especially B$_6$, magnesium, digestive enzymes, and essential fatty acids; a balanced diet free of food reactors, and a procedure to remove measle cells from Phillip's bowel, the autism diagnosis was removed by the same set of specialists who originally gave him the diagnosis. Phillip's mother now co-hosts training sessions to help parents make the necessary nutritional changes to enhance their autistic child's physical, mental, and emotional well-being.

DR. HOLK'S RX

Restoring the microflora in the gut is of utmost importance for optimal absorption. Without a healthy digestive system, many micronutrients cannot be absorbed thus causing deficiencies in certain nutrients. Supplementation of microflora (probiotics), vitamin A, vitamin B$_6$, dimethylglycine (DMG), folic acid, calcium, magnesium, essential fatty acids, tryptophan, secretin, GABA, antifungals, and digestive enzymes has shown promising results for the Autism Spectrum Disorders.

A detoxification program must also be considered but must be approached with caution as symptoms may be exacerbated during the detoxification period. Homeopathy and structural therapies (cranial sacral, massage, chiropractors, bodyworkers, etc.) as well as treatments that affect sensory processing (Sensory Integration Therapy, Auditory Integration Training, Vision Therapy, Educational Kinesiology, Son-Rise Program, etc.) all have merit and have been known to help with and/or reverse symptoms (Lemar PS, 2000).

The Autism Research Institute can refer families to a variety of books and publications to learn more about the

TABLE III. FACTORS THAT MAY PLAY A ROLE IN THE ETIOLOGY AND DEVELOPMENT OF AUTISTIC SPECTRUM DISORDERS

ENVIRONMENTAL	Lead, cadmium, aluminum, antimony, mercury, chemicals (toluene, formaldehyde, etc.)
NUTRITIONAL	Deficiency of calcium, magnesium, iron, zinc, vitamin B_6 or B_1, antioxidant, glutathione, essential fatty acid, other nutritional deficiencies
METABOLIC	Faulty liver detoxification, hypoglycemia, mold, dust, pollen, amino acid pathway abnormalities, phenosultotransferase deficiency, "renal leak" syndrome
ALLERGIC	Foods (especially gluten and casein), food coloring, artificial flavorings, additives, etc.
INTESTINAL	Leaky gut syndrome, malabsorption, candida overgrowth, incomplete protein digestion, bacterial toxins, parasite infections
IMMUNOLOGICAL	Vaccinations, viral infections

clinical options that are available to treat autism. Medical practitioners can obtain *The Clinical Options Manual* from the Autism Research Institute (*www.autism.com*), which provides the latest diagnostic methods, including testing for a wide range of possible causes of autism. A list of laboratories that conduct these tests is also included.

℀ 6 ℁

The Vaccine Macine

ARE PARENTS INFORMED REGARDING THE PROS
AND CONS OF VACCINES?

As a public health educator, I am often asked about the pros and cons of vaccinating both children and adults. Vaccines are unique in health promotion policy because they are the only products that Americans are required to take by state law. Can you imagine a state requiring an American to take a specific dosage of vitamin C daily before being allowed to enter school? When it comes to vaccinating their children, most parents don't even weigh the pros and cons for one or more reasons:

- They don't believe they have a choice in the matter.
- They believe their child's doctor wouldn't promote vaccines if they were harmful.
- They believe that the United States Government, The American Public Health Association, The Centers for Disease Control, and The Food and Drug Administration are ensuring the safety of vaccines and know vaccines are essential for promoting public health.

Most parents would be shocked to discover that:

- Federal monitoring of immunization reactions is haphazard and can't spot problems until many deaths and debilitating injuries have been reported.
- For over a decade, physicians have been required by law to discuss childhood vaccine risks and benefits in pediatric care. According to a recent study reported in *PEDIATRICS*, 40 percent of the physicians did not mention risks and 40 percent did not mention the

79

National Vaccine Injury Compensation Program (*PEDIATRICS*, 2001).

- There is little research on side effects of vaccines, when they do occur.
- There is no incentive for drug companies to produce the safest vaccines possible because they already have a captive market for their products. Minimal safety studies are done before approval of most of the vaccines used today.
- Much of the negative information regarding vaccines is withheld from the public for fear that the public will reduce their vaccine usage.
- A recent Congressional report and various lawsuits have shown that the pharmaceutical industry exerts undue influence on mandatory vaccine legislation for its own gain.
- Parents in some states do have legal means to prevent any or all vaccinations for their children if they so choose.

It is not my goal or intent to decide for any parent whether or not they should vaccinate their child. I believe that it should be the parents' decision, not the government's, their doctor's, or mine. My goal is only to impart information to help you, as parents, make an INFORMED decision about such a critical health matter. For updates on both sides of the vaccine issue, contact the National Vaccine Information Center (NVIC) at www.909shot.com.

THE RUNAWAY VACCINE TRAIN

Each state has their own laws regarding which vaccines are mandatory. The American Academy of Pediatrics and National Association of County and City Health Officials in the year 2000 recommends one Hepatitis A shot, several doses of Hepatitis B, DtaP (Diphtheria, Tetanus, Pertussis) or Tetanus-Diphtheria, Haemophilus

(Influenza type b), polio, MMR (Measles, Mumps, and Rubella), and Varicella (Chicken Pox). By the time a child enters kindergarten (or earlier if the child attends a licensed day care facility), a child will need to receive 22 or more mandatory vaccines to be considered "safely" immunized. Welcome Baby Cards from the Governors of various states and the McDonald's food chains placemats are some of the many forms of propaganda to get kids immunized. Cute cartoons of babies and toddlers saying, *Thanks for caring enough to get us immunized* (2000 McDonald's Corporation) make parents feel guilty if they aren't caught up with their child's vaccination schedule.

Each year more and more vaccines are added to the "vaccine porridge." For example, in February 2000, the FDA approved Prevnar® (by American Home Products) to prevent pneumococal disease in infants and toddlers to be given in a series of four shots at age two months, four months, six months, and 12–15 months. This company grossed $461 million dollars from the sale of this vaccine in 2000. The Centers for Disease Control (CDC) highly recommends this vaccine, which means it could become mandatory in the near future. Although strong pressure was exerted by federal officials from the CDC to recommend mandatory varicella (chicken pox) vaccinations for all children entering day care and elementary school, the mandatory requirement was voted down in some states, including Illinois, in May of 2000.

I am actually encouraged by the rash of new vaccines being pumped out annually because it has finally allowed parents to focus upon the increasing number of shots their children are being pressured to take at each well baby visit. And when certain mandatory inoculations, such as the Rotashield rotavirus are promptly removed from the market due to proven serious side effects and deaths, a red flag is being raised about how well vaccines are tested before being marketed and mandated. Following are concerns voiced by medical experts, regarding the "runaway vaccine train."

The Voice of a Medical Heretic or the Voice of a Visionary?

The late Dr. Robert S. Mendelsohn, a famous pediatrician, former official of the American Medical Association, and author of *How to Raise a Healthy Child in Spite of Your Doctor*, became a mentor of mine in 1984 when I had the privilege of receiving his undivided attention for two hours on a car trip to and from his television appearance. Although I, myself, had only been vaccinated against polio as a child in the 1950s and had an acquaintance who developed polio from taking the live polio vaccine, I never questioned the pros and cons of vaccinating my own children. It was just a routine; a part of my children's well baby visits to our pediatrician.

Dr. Mendelsohn and I both agreed wholeheartedly that allergies and nutrition, two major forces in human health, received very little attention in medical school, thus accounting for vast ignorance on the part of the medical profession. He was not surprised when I told him that our pediatrician in 1972 thought that hot dogs were a fine daily source of protein for my eldest and highly allergic son and that my son should be allowed to eat as much sugar as he desired. Until my daughter's problems began in 1974, I never questioned our pediatrician with regards to what constituted healthy foods, food reactions, or how to treat them.

When Dr. Mendelsohn then began to expound upon the biggest threat of childhood disease being caused by mass immunizations, I thought I had either been asleep at the wheel or misinterpreted his statement. But as he continued, I realized that my health belief system was about to change forever.

Dr. Mendelsohn's book, *How to Raise A Healthy Child in Spite of Your Doctor*, reiterates what he explained to me that unforgettable day in the car. These were his concerns regarding immunizations:

- There is no convincing evidence that mass immunizations eliminate childhood diseases.

- There are significant risks associated with every immunization.
- There are contraindications that may make it dangerous to immunize a child at certain times (i.e., immunizing a child when they are ill; immunizing a child with a preservative or allergen to which the child reacts).
- Neither all of the short-term nor long-term hazards of vaccines are fully known or understood. Vaccinating children is a PHILOSOPHY, not a SCIENCE.
- It is commonly believed that vaccines alone are responsible for the decline of contagious diseases, when in fact about 90 percent of these diseases were already on the decline due to other factors such as better sanitation and healthier food choices. For instance, although the Salk vaccine was thought to be responsible for halting the polio epidemic in America in the 1940s and 1950s, the epidemic also ended in Europe at the same time even though the vaccine was not widely used there.
- There is growing suspicion that immunizing children against relatively harmless diseases may be directly responsible for an increase in autoimmune diseases in adulthood.
- It is the parent, not the doctor, who needs to be the principle player in preserving a child's health. The parent(s) should make the decision as to whether their child should or should not be immunized. (Mendelsohn, 1984)

Sixteen years later, Mayer Eisenstein, M.D., M.P.H., J.D., reiterated Dr. Mendelsohn's prophetic statements in his book entitled *Safer Medicine* and on his radio shows. As more and more mandatory vaccines have entered the scene, more and more serious adverse reactions have been reported. Eisenstein has often said that much of what parents have been led to believe about immunizations simply isn't true. He not only has grave misgivings about them, but would want to urge parents to reject all vaccines if it weren't for the fact that parents in over half of the United States have lost the right to make that choice.

In *Safer Medicine*, Dr. Eisenstein reports the following "Did you know?" immunization facts:

- The Chicken Pox vaccine is grown on the tissue of aborted human babies.
- The Hepatitis B vaccine is meant to protect against Hepatitis B, a blood borne and sexually transmitted disease. Yet we give it to infants at birth.
- Vaccine recipients who receive live vaccines can transmit the disease to other individuals with whom they come into close contact.
- Live viral vaccines are contaminated with other viruses. For instance, the Live Polio Vaccine, given between 1955–1963, was contaminated with SV40 (Simian Virus). SV40 is a monkey virus that produces cancer in human beings. Could it be that the epidemic of cancers we are seeing today among baby boomers could be caused in part by the contaminated viruses from childhood vaccines?
- Vaccines may contain one or more of the following inactive ingredients:
    ethylene glycol (antifreeze)
        phenol or carbolic acid (disinfectant, dye)
        formaldehyde (an immune system suppressant and cancer-causing agent)
    aluminum (associated with Alzheimer's disease and seizures; it is an additive meant to produce an antibody response)
    thimerosal (a form of ethyl mercury used as a disinfectant/preservative; mercury is a known cause of brain injury and autoimmune disease)
    neomycin and streptomycin (antibiotics; can cause allergic reactions)

- Vaccines are grown and strained through animal or human tissues such as monkey kidney, chicken embryo, guinea pig embryonic cells, calf serum, or human diploid cells (the dissected organs of aborted fetuses as in the case of Rubella, Hepatitis A, and Chicken Pox vaccines).

- The problem with using animal cells is that animal RNA and DNA can be transferred from one host to another so that undetected animal viruses may slip into viruses injected into humans through vaccinations. What are the potential long-term effects of this? We do know for a fact that the Swine Flu vaccine of 1976 caused serious side effects, such as Guillain Barre Syndrome, paralysis, and even death.

(Eisenstein, pp. 111–35, 2000)

In a *Chicago Parent Magazine* editorial (October 2000) written by pediatrician and immunopathologist, Linda Lorincz Shelton, Ph.D., M.D., F.A.A.P., she contradicted false information regarding immunizations. Some of her comments indicate that many of Mendelsohn's prophetic statements have become true. They include the following, according to Dr. Shelton:

- *At the present time in the United States, the risk of adverse reactions to the polio vaccine is greater than the risk of contracting polio. I recommend that we stop vaccinating infants against polio.*

- *There are many unanswered questions about the long-term impact of vaccines. There has been a steady, unexplained rise in the incidence of autoimmune disease and allergic disease, such as asthma, during the vaccine era. Many scientists, including myself, believe that this may be due particularly to the measles vaccine.*

- *I believe that universal vaccination of infants with Hepatitis B vaccine will actually increase deaths from long-term consequences of chronic Hepatitis B disease, besides giving the population a false sense of security that they are immune from the disease. I ask whether a*

vaccine that is associated with 50 deaths per year and thousands of adverse events . . . is an effective shot?
- *Our civil rights should only be surrendered when the risk to society is so great as to threaten society itself. Vaccine mandates can be viewed as a form of surrendering these rights. With 300 new vaccines in the works, where will this runaway vaccine mandate train stop? The government should put more money into funding genetic research to identify those individuals who are at risk for serious adverse events when vaccinated or who will not be immune when vaccinated. This will allow us to protect those who could be harmed by vaccines.*

(Linda Lorincz Shelton, Ph.D., M.D., F.A.A.P., *Chicago Parent Magazine*, October 2000)

A SHOT IN THE DARK?

Probably, the first most publicized and eye-opening book written about the dangers of vaccines is *DPT: A Shot in the Dark* (Coulter & Fisher, 1985). This book discusses the damage caused by the DPT vaccine and vaccines in general. My concern is that parents never hear about the risks of immunizing their children until their own children suffer from debilitation or death from a vaccine. A more timely publication by *Mothering* Magazine, "Vaccination: The Issue of Our Times," is probably the most comprehensive collection of articles, research, and references challenging the convention viewpoint on vaccinations (2001). Publications like these give parents vaccine facts so that they can make informed decisions.

Here are just a few of the many cases that question the safety and efficacy of vaccines:
- The U.S. Food & Drug Administration found squalene in the Anthrax Vaccine used for Gulf War soldiers although this was a banned substance. In fact, a review by the Department of Health and Human Services found that the tainted Anthrax Vaccine

either certainly or probably caused 592 cases of Gulf War Syndrome. Were the soldiers informed that their mandatory vaccine contained the illegal use of squalene? Apparently not. Hopefully, squalene has been removed from the vaccine being recommended to individuals potentially exposed to anthrax during the recent terrorist attacks. For more information, contact *www.anthraxvaccine.org.*

- Flu shots "slightly" increase the risk of contracting a rare nerve disorder, Guillain-Barré Syndrome. "Slightly" means 60–70 cases of the disorder will occur each year. Tell this to the families of disabled or dead loved ones who were not informed of this risk before being vaccinated.

- Thimerosal-free (or mercury-free) Hepatitis B vaccines are now available due to serious reactions suffered by newborns who were given the shots. Were parents ever alerted to the fact that the vaccines contained mercury? Even my own clients find it hard to believe that vaccines could contain mercury. I tell them to insist that their children only receive mercury-free vaccines. The FDA admits that all childhood vaccines are now available in thimerosal-free versions, but are suggesting only a "phase out" over time to unload vaccine manufacturers' defective products.

According to an Autism research conference in April of 2000, it was explained that by age two, most American children receive 237 mcg. of mercury through vaccines alone. For example, the Hepatitis B, given at birth, contains 30 times the safe level; the DtaP and H:B usually given at four months contains 60 times the safe level, and the Hepatitis B and polio, usually given at six months, are 78 times the safe level. Although these toxicity levels are extremely high, **there has never been research** conducted regarding toxicity from mercury in vaccines. From the U.S. Environmental Protection Agency, we know that mercury **ingested** through food, air, and water has been associated with serious neurological disorders. In vaccines, however, mercury in the form of thimerosal is 50 times more toxic than ingested mercury. Among the reasons for this increased level of toxicity is that mercury is more toxic when injected and that infants have no blood-brain barrier to block absorption so that it accumulates in brain cells and nerves. (Bernard, Sallie. *Autism: A Unique Type of Mercury Poisoning*). What a curious coincidence that Autism was identified as a new type of mental disorder in the 1930s at the same time Thirmerosal was introduced into vaccines. Is it also a coincidence that there is a striking similarity between the symptoms of autism and mercury poisoning?

- The American Academy of Pediatrics recommended that as of January 1, 2000, all polio virus vaccines be inactivated rather than live. This change came on the wake of reports of vaccine-contracted polio from the oral polio vaccine. Were U.S. parents informed that their child's risk of getting polio from the oral polio vaccine was greater than the risk of getting polio if not vaccinated?

- The American Public Health Association (APHA) made a public plea in September 1999 to remove mercury from consumer and healthcare products on the market because they pose a serious risk of neurodevelopmental delays to fetuses and infants which can even cause cerebral palsy and mental retardation. Isn't it interesting that of all possible areas of hidden risk, the APHA never identified mercury-containing vaccines as a major player?

- Wyeth Lederle Vaccines (a division of American Home Products) voluntarily withdrew the Rotashield® rotavirus vaccine from the market in October 2000 after the Centers for Disease Control withdrew its recommendation that infants receive this vaccine to prevent diarrhea in infants and young children. It was discovered that the vaccine could cause a rare and potentially fatal bowel disorder. In fact, research has also found that it can cause Type I diabetes in some children. Why do we always find out about the serious risks created by vaccines AFTER they have been pulled off of the market? Now Wyeth Lederle has replaced the Rotashield® with their best-seller, Prevnar®. To date, 800 adverse reactions have been filed with the FDA. Prevnar® is a bio-engineered product that has never before existed on this earth. It should be interesting to see how long this vaccine will remain on the market.

- The Committee on Safety of Medicines (United Kingdom. November 2000) reported that a mass national immunization program to vaccinate all children under the age of 18 against Menigitis in 1999 has resulted in 16,000 adverse reaction, including 12 deaths, from taking the vaccines. Only 1500 people in the United Kingdom acquired the disease each year before the vaccine was available. What kind of risk vs. benefit ratio do we see here?

- The MMR (Mumps, Measles, Rubella) Vaccine used in the United Kingdom (the same one used in the United States), which was licensed in 1988, has been shown to cause several serious problems according to Andrew Wakefield, gastroenterologist at the Royal Free Hospital in London and Dr. Scott Montgomery, epidemiologist at Karolinska Hospital in Stockholm. They both have alleged that there is a correlation between the MMR vaccine and autism or severe neurological disease. Whether or not these allegations will prove true, there has been a shocking rise in autism throughout the parts of the world where many vaccines, including the MMR, are mandatory. As this book goes to press, several prestigious gastroenterology journals have reported that the measles virus has been found in the bowel of many autistic children who also suffer from inflammatory bowel disease.

- The mandatory Mumps, Measles, and Rubella (MMR) vaccine has become so controversial in the United Kingdom that it was banned in 1993 after a record number of children who were given the vaccine developed non-viral meningitis and other adverse reactions. In the United Kingdom today, the one thing the British government agrees upon, and reported in *The Journal of Adverse Drug Reactions (London) is that something needs to be done about the MMR and that there is a case to answer against the vaccine. The MMR vaccine should not have been licensed. There was not enough evidence of the safety of it to license it. The view is that the evidence was inadequate* (*The Sunday Herald*, London, December 10 and 17, 2000).

- Dr. Michele Carbone, a Loyola University Professor and contender for the Nobel Peace Prize, discovered

TABLE I: VACCINATIONS AND ADVERSE REACTIONS

Vaccine	Documented Adverse Reactions
Flu	Guillain-Barré Syndrome, neuropathy, optic neuritis, paralysis
Hepatitis B	neurological disorders, chronic fatigue syndrome, multiple sclerosis
Measles (attenuated)	middle ear infections, convulsions, tonsillitis, autoimmune disease
Measles (live)	cerebral palsy, learning disabilities, mental retardation
MMR	arthritis, autism, neurological disease
Mumps	hepatitis
Polio (oral)	contraction of polio, deafness, tinnitus
Rubella (live)	arthritis
Small pox, yellow fever, typhoid, Rabies, TB, polio polio, diptheria, tetanus	multiple sclerosis, epilepsy, death
Thermisol (mercury) containing vaccines	autism, learning disabilities, neurodevelopmental
Additive	delays

in 1994 that a virus named SV40 was found in 60 percent of all deadly human lung cancer cells as well as in some bone cancers and brain tumors. The virus, supposedly only found in monkeys, is one of the most potent human carcinogens ever discovered. It literally shuts down a cell's natural defenses against cancer. So, how did this monkey virus get into humans? **The most likely answer appears to be the SV40 tainted polio vaccine given from 1955–1963 (infecting about 30 million Americans).** The virus has to be triggered by an environmental factor for it to cause cancer. Baby boomers may have fought polio only to be threatened with a cancer time-bomb ticking away today.

It is not the scope of this book to discuss the many risks and benefits of various vaccines, although Table I gives a brief list of documented problems related to vaccines. For further enlightenment, I recommend two excellent books, *The Vaccine Guide: Making an Informed Choice* and *A Shot in the Dark*. For updates on the changing vaccine scene, I recommend contacting the National Vaccine Information Center (*www.909shot.com*).

How Vaccines are Mandated

Individual states in the United States mandate vaccines. The states say that vaccines are safe due to the expert committees (paid representatives of the drug companies) that approved them. Yet, when you review expert committee guidelines, they leave the final determination up to the state and assume absolutely no responsibility or liability for their recommendations. The drug companies that manufacture vaccines, therefore, bear little responsibility for damage caused by vaccines.

Legal red tape

If you, as well-informed parents, do decide not to vaccinate, it is important to check with your individual state to determine the law and exemptions. Each state public health department should also be able to answer questions regarding exemptions. To date, there are 42 states with mandatory vaccines and only about 17 states that grant exemptions. Most states allow limited medical exemptions and a religious exemption. A few states allow a philosophical (or conscientiously held belief) exemption. Still, it is estimated that 98 percent of American children are vaccinated.

A parent who chooses the religious exemption must submit a written and signed statement to the local school authority detailing the religious belief that conflicts with immunizations. It would be helpful if the letter is written on legal letterhead signed by an attorney. An example of such a letter for an Illinois exemption is found in Table II.

In Illinois, a licensed physician who indicates why the medical condition would preclude a child from receiving the required immunizations must make a medical exemption. I don't like this route unless your child really does have a compromised immune system, even if you can get your doctor to sign the letter. I have seen children prevented from participating in extracurricular sports when the school nurse alerted coaches about the exemption.

There is now national pressure from vaccine dissenters to get legislators to realize that forcing vaccines upon families is preventing informed consent. All of the prevailing ethical standards in medical care since World War II insist that there must be informed consent for any medical procedure that carries a risk of injury or death. It has been proven over and over again that vaccines carry this risk. Why, then, have they been excluded from informed consent?

The door is definitely open for *thinking clearly about the ramifications of forced immunization for the public.* In October 2000, members of the Association of American Physicians and Surgeons (AAPS) voted unanimously to put a moratorium on vaccine mandates and for physicians to insist upon truly informed consent before vaccinating. The group insists that this is **not** a vote against vaccines, but that the rights of the parents, and each individual child's needs must be looked at medically without the forced hand of the government. Due to roughly 11,000 cases of reactions following vaccines reported annually, Dr. Jane Orient, a spokesman for AAPS, made this comment: *Our children face the possibility of death or serious long-term adverse effects from mandated vaccines that aren't necessary or that have very limited benefits.* AAPS believes

---

TABLE II: LEGAL SCHOOL VACCINATION AND IMMUNIZATION EXEMPTION

School Name: _____

School Address: _____

Student Name: _____

Student Address: _____

THE LEGAL PARENT: _____ states the above child is HEREBY EXEMPT from immunizations on RELIGIOUS GROUNDS of the ILLINOIS COMPILED STATUTES, Chapter 105, Section 5/27-8.1, Subsection (8), since it is in conflict with the parents bona fide sincere held beliefs and practices of their religious faith, which violate the natural laws of health put forth within them by a higher force of creation, by introducing unnecessary toxins which destroy the natural built-in immunity that is already present in a healthy body. This document fulfills the requirements of the 77 ILLINOIS ADMINISTRATIVE CODE, Chapter I, Subchapter I, Subpart E, Section 665-510.

The above exemption was approved August 13, 1979, by Governor James Thompson, House Bill 2301 State of Illinois.

According to the ILLINOIS DEPARTMENT OF HEALTH, Springfield, objection to immunization is not required on Church letterhead or executed by an official of any church or denomination.

The above LEGAL PARENT assumes FULL RESPONSIBILITY for their child's health, thus removing same from school as far as the vaccines go.

THIS LETTER IS LEGAL-TO BE FILED WITH STUDENT'S HEALTH RECORD.

_____

LEGAL and VALID SIGNATURE OF PARENT

that parents, with the advice of their doctors, should make decisions about their children's medical care – not government bureaucrats. (AAPS, 57th Annual Meeting, St. Louis, MO, October 2000). I say bravo for this group of doctors who have the courage to try to change the status quo. I feel it is only a matter of time before other physicians groups adopt the same position. How can they do less when our medical freedom is at stake? Nichola McCutcheon, 20-months-old, died eight hours after a reaction to his DPT shot. Julie Middlehurst-Schwartz suffered her first grand mal seizure within hours of her DPT shot at four-months-old. She died from an epileptic seizure at the age of three. These children *had no voice . . . they had no choice*. This should never happen to another child. (DPT®Dissatisfied Parents Together).

THE MISSING ELEMENT: A HEALTHY IMMUNE SYSTEM

Dr. Thomas Stone, an M.D., member of the American Board of Environmental Medicine, and Diplomat of the American Board of Psychiatry and Neurology, feels that few, if any, complications of contracting childhood diseases arise in parts of the world where healthy food is consumed and immunological functions of the child are sufficient. In fact, most generations before polio in the United States remember getting all of the childhood diseases. The children stayed home from school a few days, received extra pampering, and returned to school, proud that their immune systems had been challenged and won. It was unheard of to hear of classmates being hospitalized or permanently impaired after contracting measles, mumps, rubella, whooping cough, or chicken pox. In fact, having a child's immune system challenged early in life has been shown repeatedly to ward off many autoimmune diseases later in life. Dr. Stone emphasized that the real solution for preventing or effectively fighting childhood infections is the development of an intact, functioning immune system developed through adequate nutrition ("Vaccines," NOHA Newsletter, 1992).

Dr. Lendon Smith, a famous pediatrician, reiterates Dr. Stone's comments. He said in his March 4, 1994, newsletter, *with proper nutrients, we all . . . can attain an optimum level of health with our own white blood cells and immunoglobins despite bad genes* ("Are We Kidding Ourselves?", *The Facts*, March 1994).

Childhood illnesses of former times (mumps, rubella, chicken pox, measles) entered the body through the mucous membranes. These minor illnesses had a positive purpose in challenging and strengthening the immune system. In contrast, their respective vaccines are injected by needle directly into a child's system bypassing the mucous membranes. As a result, immune systems of many children remain relatively weak and stunted because they have never been challenged. At least four controlled studies (Incao, 1997; Sheneen, *Lancet*, 1996; Odnet, *JAMA*, 1999, and Kemp, *Epidemolgy*, 1997) have confirmed that complications from failing to challenge the immune system may be implicated in the rapid rise in frequency and severity of asthma and eczema.

Imagine what would happen if the United States used the money now earmarked for free or reduced cost vaccination programs to provide free vitamin, mineral, and nutrient-dense foods to children living in impoverished areas. Not only would we see healthier kids, but we would also see kids better able to cope in life physically, mentally, emotionally, and socially. It is also important to note that as far back as 1995, a promising development in vaccine research indicated that harmless proteins can trigger an immune response in the body that can eliminate adverse reactions to vaccines (*TIME Magazine*, January 23, 1995). Why hasn't this research been put into practice and why hasn't the public heard more about this new technology?

COVERING ALL BASES

After thoroughly researching the vaccine subject, many parents will still opt to vaccinate their children. With their newfound knowledge, however, they will want to take every precaution to ensure more benefit than risk with immunizations. Following is a list of recommendations to ensure the highest standard of vaccine safety:

- **Delay all vaccines until your child's immune system is developed.** *The Vaccine Guide: Making An Informed Choice* recommends delaying the initiation of vaccines until a child's immune system is fully developed, usually by 24 months of age. Delaying the initiation of vaccines until then will not reduce their effectiveness. The reason for recommending vaccines during the first year of life evolved out of convenience because doctors have more access to children in the first year of life at well baby visits.

- **Do not vaccinate your child with more than one vaccine at a time**. Combining vaccines is only given out of convenience, not necessity. The effectiveness of one vaccine may be hampered by another. Also, the risk of compromising the immune system increases with the more vaccines that are given simultaneously. Especially avoid giving a viral with a bacterial vaccination (i.e., MMR with pneumococcus). The development of a "super vaccine" is in the works. The consequences of this may be devastating. You may have to see your child's doctor every month for a year, but it is worth it to vaccinate slowly.

- **Do not vaccinate your child when he or she is ill**. A runny nose, a cough, or especially being on an antibiotic for an infection, should prevent your physician from even offering to vaccinate. Unfortunately, many doctors will still opt to vaccinate, with potentially devastating consequences (see this chapter's Case Study).

- **The day before, day of, and day after any vaccine, protect your child's immune system by administering vitamins and minerals.** Dr. Lendon Smith and other preventive physicians recommend the following dosages: 100–500 mg. of Vitamin C (100 mg. if one year old, 250 mg. if 18 months, and

500 mg. if two-years or older), 10–50 mg. of B-6 (10 mg. if one year old, 25 mg. if 18 months, and 50 mg. if two years or older), 250–500 mg. of extra calcium and 175–250 mg. of extra magnesium (250 mg. calcium with 125 mg. magnesium from 12–24 months, 500 mg. calcium with 250 mg. magnesium if 25 months or older). If the child appears feverish or ill in any way, continue the regimen until the symptoms subside and contact your physician immediately. Don't be a "vaccine guinea pig."

- **Unless a vaccine is mandatory, avoid it.** With 300 new vaccines in the works, the "runaway vaccine train" has to stop somewhere. Also, avoid any new vaccine, unless mandatory, if it has not been on the market at least two years. Many vaccines are taken off within that time period due to devastating side effects.

- **Insist that your child's vaccine be thimerosal (mercury)-free and free of any of your child's known allergens.** Insist that your child's physician or drug manufacturer provide you with additive information. It is a shame that most doctors don't routinely volunteer this information.

- If your child's physician pushes to immunize earlier than you desire or you opt not to have your child be immunized at all, tell the doctor you will be more than happy to immunize if the doctor will sign a Vaccine Pledge (see Table III for an example). I can't tell you how quickly your doctor will "let you off the hook" rather than being asked to explain why she won't sign the pledge.

- If your child or someone you know may have suffered a vaccine injury, please contact the Williams Bailey Law Firm in Houston, Texas, for more information regarding how to file a lawsuit for vaccine-related injuries (1-888-709-6674). For suspected vaccine toxicity from mercury (thimerosal) exposure, contact the law firm of Waters & Kraus and ask for Victoria Gibson at 1-800-226-9880.

TABLE III: VACCINE PLEDGE

I, Dr. _____, do solemnly swear that the vaccine(s) I am about to administer to (name of child) have been tested for safety by their respective drug manufacturers. I also swear that the vaccine(s) does not contain any mercury, formaldehyde, aluminum, or other known toxins.

I have also explained possible long-term risks vs. benefits of the vaccine(s) I am about to administer to the parent(s). The child shows no signs of illness at this time.

_____   _____
Physician   Child's Parent

_____
Date

Parents have the responsibility to provide the best health care possible for their own children. It should be your decision, based upon research and risk vs. benefit information, to decide whether or not to vaccinate or how to best vaccinate your children. A child who dies from a vaccine is just as important as a child who dies from an infectious disease. Hopefully, your child's physician will honor your decisions regarding vaccinations. If not, it is time to look for a more knowledgeable, open-minded doctor.

Personal Case Study #6

A mother brought in her seven-year-old identical twins. Justin R. sat in my waiting room reading a book and doing homework. Jake R. was the child the mother had concerns about. He was severely mentally delayed, hyperkinetic, and agitated. His speech was slurred and his behavior was on the par of a typical three-year-old. He exhibited many food and drug reactions. The mother was hoping that certain vitamins, minerals, and nutrient-dense foods could improve her child's chances of leading a more normal life. He was now attending all special classes and was shuttled from therapist to therapist.

Before I gave my recommendations, she wanted me to know how her son became brain damaged. Both of her twins had developed normally until the age of eighteen months. At that time, she brought them in for their eighteen-month check-up, where they were scheduled to receive MMR, Polio, and DTP vaccines. Justin was well. Jake was on the last day of an antibiotic for an ear infection. The mother even told her pediatrician that she would bring Jake back in a few weeks when he was healthier, but the doctor insisted that the ear infection was most certainly cleared up and that it would be okay to vaccinate.

The evening of receiving the vaccines, Jake spiked a high fever, went into convulsions, and became "almost a vegetable" for weeks. The mischievous sparkle left his eyes, and the family has spent the last 5½ years slowly trying to "bring him back." The family doesn't know if it was the vaccine, the antibiotic, the combination of the vaccine and antibiotic, or Jake's weakened immune system, but they do know Jake should never have received one vaccine, let alone three on that day. Yes, the mother is angry with her doctor for pressuring her, but she is angrier with herself for allowing herself to be pressured when she violated her motherly instincts. She now has become an expert on vaccines and has chosen not to vaccinate anyone in her family ever again.

DR. HOLK'S RX: HOMEOPATHIC "VACCINATIONS"

Homeopathy historically came into popularity due to its therapeutic success in the treatment of epidemics. In the 1800s outbreaks of diseases, such as cholera and yellow fever, claimed many lives. The use of homeopathy was so impressive that a board of conventional medical doctors for the United States Government actually published a report discussing the successful treatment of yellow fever with homeopathy (Coulter H, 1973). By the turn of the century, with the rise of penicillin, the focus of medicine turned to drugs and the use of homeopathy declined in the United States. Other parts of the world, however, still used homeopathy and acknowledged its therapeutic importance.

Since homeopathy rose to stardom with its successful use in the care of epidemics, it is theorized that homeopathy may offer an alternative form of "vaccination." By giving a child a homeopathic preparation from diseased tissue or secretions that is diluted and succussed many times over, a sharpened immune response may result to that particular organism. Since there are no physical antigens being injected into the body, it is highly unlikely that a physical antibody immune response will be evoked. What may occur, however, is an energetic fine-tuning of the immune system. From my perspective as a biophysics instructor, I recognize that the explanation of how homeopathy works lies in the realm of quantum physics. Once these principles are applied to homeopathy, I am sure the energetics of homeopathy will come to light!

As a naturopathic physician, however, I would not currently recommend that homeopathy be given in place of an immunization. I do strongly advocate educating yourself, as a parent, about the **risks and benefits** of vaccines. Talk to many practitioners and have your child's vital energy evaluated. There are some children who simply do not have enough vital energy to effectively surmount the dramatic stress placed on their immature immune system. Proper timing of immunizations is imperative. If you decide to vaccinate, the use of homeopathy after each vaccination can be extremely helpful in clearing some of the residual after effects of the vaccines. Please consult with a homeopathic physician for individual recommendations

≈℃ 7 ℈≈

Osteoporosis Begins in Childhood

Osteoporosis is not often associated with children but has become an important pediatric concern. Bone mass is built during the first three decades of life and peaks between the ages of 30 and 35 years. Children and young adults who are unable to build peak bone mass during this time predispose themselves to fractures throughout life and osteoporosis later in life.

WHAT CAUSES OSTEOPOROSIS?

How and why osteoporosis occurs is not fully understood. However, risk factors for the disease have been identified and are outlined in Table I.

MAJOR PLAYERS IN BONE HEALTH

Calcium is an essential mineral that plays an important role in bone health, muscular contraction, glandular secretion, and nerve conduction. The body regulates calcium levels in the blood (serum calcium) very closely. When serum calcium levels are low, the body restores proper blood levels by pulling calcium from the bones. If this process continues, the bones lose their density and strength because the breakdown of bone exceeds the building of bone. A diet high in refined sugar, fat, phosphates, and salt may actually rob calcium from bones as does alcohol abuse and cigarette smoking.

Phosphorus is as essential to bone health as is calcium. Phosphorus is very abundant in our diets, which means we usually get too much of it, almost double the amount we need each day. The **right** amount of phosphorus

promotes absorption of calcium while too much acceler-
ates calcium loss.

Soft drinks not only contain phosphorus, but also sugar
and caffeine, all of which leach calcium from bone. A
study of teenagers measured their urinary calcium loss
after drinking soft drinks with or without caffeine and
sugar. Results showed that urinary calcium levels increased
from 6 mg to 20 mg per hour with the ingestion of the caffeinated drink. Urinary calcium excretion increased from
16 mg to 30 mg per hour after ingestion of the soft drink
with both caffeine and sugar. Urinary excretion of other
important electrolytes such as sodium, potassium, and
chloride increased as well (Massey LK., 1988).

Magnesium plays an extremely important role in the
absorption of calcium. Magnesium is essential for over
300 metabolic reactions in the body. It is important for
the normal functioning of the parathyroid glands and in
the metabolism of vitamin D, both of which play an
important role in calcium homeostasis. A deficiency of
magnesium can produce a wide variety of symptoms
including neuromuscular problems, gastrointestinal
upset, cardiovascular abnormalities, and disrupted calcium homeostasis.

Vitamin D helps to maintain blood calcium levels within an acceptable range. The term "vitamin" is actually
misleading. Vitamin D is really a hormone that is found
in the skin and activated by a complex set of reactions
that require ultraviolet radiation, namely sunlight. A
deficiency of vitamin D results in defective mineraliza-
tion of the skeleton leading to permanent bone deformities. This pathology, when seen in children is called
rickets and, when seen in adults is called osteomalacia.
Historically, rickets was noted as early as 1650 but it was-
n't until the late 1800s when scientists realized the role
that sunlight and vitamin D played in correcting this
condition. As a result, in the 1930s, the United States and
Europe began fortifying foods with vitamin D to help
prevent a deficiency. Because of this, rickets has been

TABLE I. FACTORS COMMONLY ASSOCIATED WITH OSTEOPOROSIS

Nutritional factors

Lifelong low dietary calcium ,
  magnesium, zinc and vitamin D
  intake
Milk intolerance and allergy
Excessive alcohol intake
Excess phosphorus intake, especially
  from soft drinks

Lifestyle

Inactivity, especially lack of weight-
  bearing activities
Smoking
Nulliparity (not having given birth)
Excess exercise (producing amenor-
  rhea, i.e., loss of menstruation)
Early natural menopause
Late menarche

Drugs

Thyroid replacement drugs
Glucocorticoid drugs
Anticoagulants (heparin)
Chronic lithium therapy
Gonadotropin releasing hormone
  agonist or antagonist therapy
Anticonvulsant drugs
Extended tetracycline use*
Diuretics producing calciuria*

Genetic

White or Asiatic ethnicity
Positive family history
Small body frame (less than 58 kg)

Medical disorders

Anorexia nervosa
Cushing's syndrome
Diabetes?Type 1
Thyrotoxicosis
Alterations in gastrointestinal and
  hepatobiliary function
Occult osteogenesis imperfecta
Mastocytosis
Rheumatoid arthritis
Long-term parenteral nutrition
Prolactinoma
Hemolytic anemia, hemochromatosis,
  and thalassemia
Ankylosing spondylitis
Phenonthiazine derivatives*
Cyclosporin*
Aluminum-containing antacids*

---

* Not yet associated with decreased bone
mass although identified as either toxic to
bone in animals or inducing calciuria
and/or calcium malabsorption in human
beings.

Adapted from Dempster DW and Lindsay R. "Pathogenesis of Osteoporosis." *Lancet.*
341:800, 1993.

---

considered an eradicated disease process. However, with
the concerns about skin cancer and the increased use of
sunscreens that block the ultraviolet radiation of the sun
from the skin, rickets is once again on the rise, especially
among young children.

Twenty minutes in the sun daily with face and arms
exposed will synthesize the recommended daily allowance
of vitamin D. The best times during the day are morning or

late afternoon when the sun is not directly overhead. Allow your child to have these few minutes without sunscreen. Depending on where you live, getting enough sunlight in the winter months may be difficult. If this is the case, a great dietary supplement for getting adequate vitamin D and strengthening the immune system is cod liver oil, in liquid or capsule form (see Chapter 14 for specific details).

Boron reduces calcium secretion. Low levels are often found in patients who have osteoporosis.

Protein balance affects bone health. While it has been shown that too much protein, especially from red meat, can cause an increased loss of calcium in the urine, too little protein can have disastrous consequences as well. Protein helps to build new tissue, including bone. Children who avoid protein may never build strong bones. This will put them at a much higher risk for osteoporosis in adulthood.

COULD WE BE GETTING TOO MUCH OF A GOOD THING?

A number of researchers today are becoming "dairy doubters" because the countries where the most cow's milk is consumed have the highest levels of hip fractures. Could the problem be too much calcium? In countries, where the intake of calcium comes from green leafy vegetables and is half of what is recommended in the United States, the incidence of hip fracture is up to one-fifth that of the United States. Some researchers theorize that getting too much calcium may actually decrease the amount of the mineral that is absorbed by excreting the excess. With less supply from the diet, the efficiency with which calcium is absorbed and utilized may increase.

WHAT'S THE BEST WAY TO GET CALCIUM?

Consuming bioavailable calcium in supplement form and increasing **non-dairy**, calcium-rich foods is important. Table II highlights the calcium content of some non-diary foods.

TABLE II. Calcium Content of Foods* (Non-dairy Choices)

Food Item	Calcium (mg.)	Food Item	Calcium (mg.)
Almonds (1/2 cup)	160	Parsley (1 cup)	80
Blackberries (1/2 cup)	45	Peanuts (1/2 cup)	110
Bok Choy (1 cup)	250	Pecans (1/2 cup)	40
Broccoli (1 cup)	40	Salmon, canned pink (4 oz.)	220
Brussel sprouts (1 cup)	50	Salmon, canned red (4 oz.)	290
Cabbage (1 cup)	35	Sardines, canned with bones	
Carrots (1 cup)	45	(4 oz.)	500
Celery pieces (1 cup)	40	Scallops, fresh (4 oz.)	130
Collard Greens (1 cup)	290	Seaweed, hijiki (1/2 cup)	300
Corn tortilla, lime-treated (3.5 oz.)	300	Shrimp, fresh (4 oz.)	130
Dandelion greens (1 cup)	205	Soybeans, cooked (1 cup)	140
Haddock (3 oz.)	210	Spinach, raw (1 cup)	200
Kale (1 cup)	150	Squash, cooked (1 cup)	55
Kidney beans (1 cup)	75	Sunflower seeds, raw (1/2 cup)	65
Lima beans (1 cup)	65	Sweet potatoes, cooked (1 cup)	50
Milk substitutes (1 cup)**	200–300	Tilapia, fresh farm-raised (4 oz.)	120
Mackerel, canned (4 oz.)	300	Tofu (4 oz.)	145
Mustard greens (1 cup)	60	Tofu, enriched (4 oz.)	280
Tuna, oil-packed (3 oz.)	200	Turnip greens (1 cup)	250
Navy beans (1 cup)	100	Walnuts (1/2 cup)	50
Orange (1 medium)	55	Watercress (1 cup)	40
Orange juice (calcium fortified)	300		

*The amounts of calcium listed above are approximations; organically grown items may contain more calcium and overly processed foods may contain less.
**For a list of milk substitutes, see "Non-Dairy Milk Substitutes."

Source: *Bowes & Church's Food Values of Portions Commonly Used,* Jean A. Pennington, 1998

Supplementing with calcium can be beneficial, if the calcium is lead-free and highly absorbable (oyster shell and bone meal calcium sources have been shown to contain high levels of lead). Calcium carbonate will almost always be malabsorbed by the elderly and those with low stomach acid due to its antacid effect. Calcium carbonate interferes with protein digestion and can cause gas, bloating, and constipation. Calcium bound to citrate, fumarate, glycinate, malate, succinate and aspartate are recommended as the best absorbed forms. They may, however, fail to build bone effectively because they are not a complete bone food. Microcrystalline Hydroxyapatite Concentrate (MCHC), the most complete bone food that is free of toxic substances, is well absorbed and has been shown repeatedly to reduce bone loss and restore lost bone. MCHC provides much greater nourishment than does calcium alone. It contains protein and other ingredients that comprise the organic portion of bone, as well as calcium and other minerals in the normal physiological proportions found in raw bone. Numerous case studies of individuals switching from heavy dairy product intake and/or incomplete bone food supplements to MCHC have seen evidence of rapid restoration of broken bones and improvements in significant bone density (3–7 percent per year), even among osteoporotic females.

It is important to note that the gateway to proper absorption of calcium is the stomach where calcium is solubilized and ionized. Stomach acid is essential for absorption of calcium. Children and/or young adults who are or have been on continuous steroid drugs are susceptible to low stomach acid. Low stomach acid, or hypochlorhydria, has been shown to adversely affect the absorption of calcium. Because of malabsorption issues, hypochlorhydrics have a higher risk of getting osteoporosis than do individuals in the normal population.

BONE ROBBERS

Table III gives some general information about common "bone robbers" and other dietary factors that cause calcium loss. It is impossible to build or maintain bone if calcium is continuously being excreted.

ACID AS AN UNRECOGNIZED CAUSE OF OSTEOPOROSIS

Dr. Susan Lark, MD, one of the foremost authorities in the fields of clinical nutrition and preventive medicine, researched studies back to the 1930s that confirmed diet as instrumental in bone health. She states that acid/base balance of our blood is the key to proper bone health. Blood pH should be slightly alkaline. However, the

TABLE III. BONE ROBBERS	
Too Much Sodium	An excess of 2000 mg. consumed daily contributes to increased calcium excretion (loss in the urine).
Too Much Vitamin A	Too much vitamin A can block calcium absorption. This is of particular concern for female teens taking vitamin A prescriptions for acne problems. Tetracycline, another often-prescribed medication for acne, increases urinary calcium excretion.
Too Much Phosphorus	Too much phosphorus (highly processed foods, red meat, and soft drinks) can bind calcium and excrete it from the body.
Mineral Imbalances	Imbalances of magnesium, calcium, phosphorus, zinc, and boron can contribute to poor bone health.
Antacid Calcium Supplements	Antacid calcium sources are less than ideal calcium supplements because gastric acid is necessary for calcium absorption.
Low Stomach Acid	Inhibits proper calcium breakdown and absorption. Important to consider with long-term steroid drug therapy, lack of B_{12} (necessary to produce stomach acid), and hypochlorhydria.
Too Much Insoluble Fiber	(whole wheat, psyllium, phytates in beans) Can block calcium absorption. Ideally, calcium and high fiber foods should be consumed at separate times.
Too Much Caffeine	Too much coffee or excess caffeine (more than three cups of caffeinated coffee daily) causes calcium excretion.

Sources: Lark S. "Beautiful Bone-Part I." *The Lark Letter.* 8(5), 2001.
Marz, Russell, N.D. Medical Nutrition from Marz. 2nd ed., Portland, Oregon: Omni-Press, 1997.
Murray MT. "Osteoporosis prevention and treatment-beyond calcium." Natural Medicine Journal 1999;2(5):5-12.
Pizzorno JE and Murray MT. Textbook of Natural Medicine, 2nd edition, London: Churchill Lange. 1991.

American diet supplies more acidic foods causing the pH to be more acidic. As the body tries to neutralize an acid-diet rich in red meat, dairy, sugar products and alcohol, alkalizing agents like calcium and magnesium are being overused. Cow's milk products create excess acid. The body eventually pulls calcium from the bone to maintain proper acid-base balance. The American Diet is very high in acid, which is one reason why we have the second highest rate of osteoporosis worldwide. Dr. Lark recommends an alkalizing diet which includes low acid fruits, vegetables, and whole eggs (*The Lark Letter*, May 2001). For details regarding acid/alkaline foods, see Chapter 14.

Personal Case Study #7

Jacob and his parents came to see me to determine if nutritional support could reduce their son's bone loss and recurrence of kidney stones. At age thirteen, Jacob had been diagnosed with osteoporosis, which did not respond to bone-building medication. Jacob was also very short for his age and had not grown in over a year.

I felt very strongly that Jacob was suffering from Celiac Disease (genetic gluten intolerance), which was later confirmed by a pediatric gastroenterologist. His inability to digest his diet of bagels, whole grain cereals, cakes, and cookies was causing malabsorption. He also ate large doses of chocolate and spinach (high oxalate foods) and suffered from severe lactose intolerance. Both can lead to osteoporosis and kidney stones in predisposed individuals.

Alkalizing Jacob's body with fruits and vegetables while avoiding gluten, chocolate, and cow's milk foods was quite a challenge for the family. The addition of digestive enzymes, a multiple vitamin/mineral high in vitamin B_6, magnesium, zinc, and moderate calcium allowed Jacob to grow three inches the following year. Two years later, he has shown gain in bone density and no new kidney stones.

DR. HOLK'S RX: ALKALIZE YOUR BODY

Each cell requires a very stable environment in order to live. Cells exhibit the same characteristics of life that we do. They move, grow, respond to their environment, breathe, reproduce, as well as absorb, digest, assimilate foodstuffs, and excrete waste products. All of these processes occur in a watery environment that is maintained at a slightly alkaline pH. The pH of a solution is an indicator of the amount of hydrogen or hydroxyl ions in solution. When hydrogen ions predominate, the solution is said to be acidic. When hydroxyl ions predominate, the solution is alkaline. All of the metabolic processes that occur in the body do so most efficiently in an alkaline environment.

When our children consume a diet that is acid-forming, their bodies are required to neutralize the acid by sequestering alkalizing agents. Two of the agents that can help in this process are calcium and magnesium. When there are not enough of these minerals available in the blood, the body will draw upon its alkalizing calcium and magnesium reserves in the bone, robbing the bone of the material it needs to be strong and healthy.

~⫘ 8 ⫘~

Eating Disorders and Obesity

WHAT IS AN EATING DISORDER?

According to the Center for Eating Disorders at St. Joseph Medical Center in Towson, Maryland, *eating disorders include a range of conditions that involve an obsession with food, weight and appearance to the degree that a person's health, relationships and daily activities are adversely affect-ed. Whether a person restricts food intake, binge-eats, binges and purges, abuses laxatives, compulsively overeats or exces-sively exercises, these behaviors often are symptoms and not the problem* (St. Joseph Medical Center, *http://www.eating-disorders.com/whatis.htm, 2001*). It is important to realize that, as stated by the National Institute of Mental Health (NIMH), eating disorders are not due to a failure of will or behavior. They are real, treatable, medical illnesses where certain maladaptive patterns of eating take on a life of their own (NIMH, Publication No. 01-4901, 2001). Factors that may place a person at risk for eating disor-ders include genetics, stress, trauma, environmental factors, family dynamics, inadequate coping skills, nutri-ent deficiencies and food sensitivities leading to food addictions.

TYPES OF EATING DISORDERS AND THEIR SYMPTOMS

There are two main types of eating disorders: anorexia nervosa and bulimia nervosa. The common symptoms for each disorder are listed in Table I.

Binge-eating disorder is a third type of eating disorder which has no formal diagnostic criteria but is recognized by recurrent episodes of binging that occur, on an average, at least two days a week for six months (DSM-IV, 1994).

TABLE I. SYMPTOMS OF EATING DISORDERS

Anorexia Nervosa Symptoms	Bulimia Nervosa Symptoms
Resistance to maintaining body weight at or above a minimally normal weight for age and height	Recurrent episodes of binge eating, characterized by eating an excessive amount of food within a distinct period of time and by a sense of lack of control over eating during the episode
Intense fear of gaining weight or becoming fat even though underweight	Recurrent inappropriate compensatory behavior in order to prevent weight gain, such as self-induced vomiting or misuse of laxatives, diuretics, enemas or other medications (purging), fasting or excessive exercise
Disturbance in the way in which one's body weight or shape is experienced, undue influence of body weight or shape on self-evaluation, or denial of the seriousness of the current low body weight	Binge eating and inappropriate compensatory behaviors both occur on average at least twice a week for three months
Infrequent or absent menstrual periods (in females who have reached puberty)	Self-evaluation is unduly influenced by body shape and weight

Source: National Institute of Mental Health. *Eating Disorders: Facts About Eating Disorders and the Search for Solutions.* Publication No. 01-4901. Rockville, MD: NIMH, 2001.

Binge eating is defined as eating an amount of food that is definitely larger than most people would eat during a similar period of time (e.g., within a two-hour period) and under similar circumstances. A sense of lack of control over eating during the episode (e.g., a feeling that one cannot stop eating or control what or how much one is eating) is exhibited. Binge eating is not associated with the regular use of inappropriate compensatory behaviors (e.g., purging, fasting, excessive exercise) and does not occur exclusively during the course of anorexia nervosa or bulimia nervosa. Marked distress about binge eating is common. Three or more of the following criteria must be present for the disorder to be considered (NIMH, Publication No. 01-4901, 2001):

- eating much more rapidly than normal
- eating until feeling uncomfortably full
- eating large amounts of food when not feeling physically hungry
- eating alone because of being embarrassed by how much one is eating
- feeling disgusted with oneself, depressed, or very guilty after overeating

EATING DISORDERS AND THEIR EFFECTS

If your child has an eating disorder, she may also be experiencing a wide range of emotions including depression, feelings of shame, guilt, low self-esteem, perfectionism and/or negative thoughts. Sometimes children show an "all-or-nothing mentality." They may withdraw and/or have impaired relationships with family and friends. Physiological effects of eating disorders can pose grave medical risks. Symptoms can be mild at first but eventually lead to serious medical complications and in some cases, even death. Table II lists the physical effects of bulimia, anorexia, and binge eating disorder with the signs and symptoms your health practitioner will look for to determine if your child has an eating disorder.

HOW CONCERNED SHOULD I BE FOR MY CHILD IF I SUSPECT THAT MY CHILD HAS AN EATING DISORDER?

More than five million Americans experience eating disorders. Three percent of adolescent and adult women and one percent of men have anorexia nervosa, bulimia nervosa, or a binge-eating disorder (NIMH, *Eating Disorders*, 1994). A young woman with anorexia is 12 times more likely to die in comparison to non-anorexic women her age (Sullivan PF, 1995). Fifteen percent of young women have substantially disordered eating

TABLE II. PHYSICAL EFFECTS OF EATING DISORDERS

Anorexia Nervosa	Bulimia Nervosa	Binge-Eating
Fainting spells	Bloodshot eyes	Overweight/obesity
Hair loss	Tooth and gum erosion	Hyperlipidemia (increased risk of)
Diminished thyroid activity (slow metabolism, reflexes, cold hands and feet)	Sore throat	Diabetes Type II (increased risk of)
Irregular heartbeat, slow heart rhythm (can lead to cardiac arrest)	Electrolyte imbalance (which can lead to irregular heartbeat and cardiac arrest)	Cardiovascular disease/ Heart attack (increased risk of)
Low blood pressure	Heartburn/indigestion	Stroke (increased risk of due to obesity)
Decreased growth of body hair	Swollen glands in neck and face	Hypertension (increased risk of)
Dry skin	Kidney, liver and bowel damage	Degenerative Joint Disease (increased risk of)
Brittle bones and nails; bone loss	Skin rashes	Certain cancers: colon, rectum, and prostate in males; tract, breast, and ovary in females (increased risk for)
For teenagers, slowed growth/development, short stature	Enlarged parotid gland	Digestive tract diseases such as gallstones and gastric reflux problems (increased risk of)
Loss of menstruation	Intestinal ulcers	
Swollen joints	Bloating	
Infertility	Irregular menstruation	
Dehydration	Dehydration	
Dangerously low blood pressure	Dangerously low blood pressure	
Dangerously low body temperature		

Source: American Anorexia Bulimia Association
National Association of Anorexia Nervosa and Associated Disorders
National Center for Health Statistics
Tierney LM, McPhee SJ, Papadakis MA. *Current Medical Diagnosis & Treatment.*
    2000. p. 1222.

TABLE III. DANGER SIGNS FOR EATING DISORDERS

Anorexia Nervosa	Bulimia Nervosa
Preoccupation with food, weight and body	Binge eating, usually in secret
Refusal to eat, except for tiny portions	Vomiting after a binge
Continuing to diet, although thin	Frequent trips to the bathroom after meals
Abnormal weight loss	Abusing laxatives, diuretics, diet pills or emetics
Weakness, exhaustion	Weakness, exhaustion
Compulsive exercise	Compulsive exercise

Source: National Association of Anorexia Nervosa and Associated Disorders
American Anorexia Bulimia Association
National Center for Health Statistics

attitudes and behaviors (Mintz LB, Betz NE, 1988). Between 10 percent and 15 percent of those diagnosed with bulimia nervosa are men (Andersen AE, Holman JE, 1977). Forty percent of fourth graders report that they diet either "very often" or "sometimes" (Gustafson-Larson A, Terry RD, 1992). With these sobering statistics, it is important to observe your child for any change in eating habits. Table III lists the "danger signs" to look for. Seek professional help if you suspect a problem.

HOW ARE EATING DISORDERS TREATED?

Eating disorders can be treated successfully. A comprehensive evaluation of your child by a qualified professional health practitioner is an important first step. Most eating disorders are treated in outpatient settings. A combination of therapies may be used including individual psychotherapy, group psychotherapy, nutritional counseling, family psychotherapy and, if indicated, medication (NIMH, 2001). There are many levels of treatment available, ranging from intensive outpatient programs to partial and 24-hour hospitalization programs. Here are

some local and national programs to contact for immediate information and assistance:

- EDAP® Eating Disorders Awareness and
  Prevention; (800) 931-2237, *www.edap.org*
- Northwestern Medical Center, Chicago, Illinois;
  (312) 695-2269
- University of Illinois at Chicago Medical Center,
  Chicago, Illinois; (312) 996-2200
- Center for Eating Disorder-St. Joseph Medical
  Center, Towson, Maryland 21204-7582;
  (410) 427-2100; *www.eating-disorders.com*
- Harvard Eating Disorder Centers; 356 Boylston
  Street, Boston, Massachusetts 02116;
  (617) 236-7766; *www.hedc.org*

NUTRITIONAL SUPPORT FOR EATING DISORDERS

I have never counseled an individual with an eating disorder who was not deficient in at least two minerals and
at least one B-vitamin (this usually includes zinc, magnesium, iron, B_6, B_{12}, and folic acid).

Psychological therapy is not usually effective unless
these deficiencies are corrected because all of these nutrients dramatically affect emotions. A well-formulated
multi-vitamin and mineral supplement containing the
Recommended Daily Intake (RDI) for all minerals and at
least 50 mg. of B_6, 400 mcg. of folic acid, and 200 mcg. of
B_{12} can show dramatic behavioral improvements among
teens and adults. Zinc, in particular, is essential for stimu-
lating the appetite of anorexics and calming the "urge to
purge" bulimics. Zinc helps with all eating disorders
because it gives appropriate signals for hunger and fullness.

It is very important for anorexics to see a nutrition
counselor weekly if their weight becomes dangerously
low so that weigh-ins are routine and small amounts of
food can be added slowly. When an anorexic child or
teen becomes aware that hospitalization will be required

if their weight drops below a certain number, they usually will have better accountability.

PROMISING NEW THERAPIES

The Maudsley approach is a promising method of working with early-onset, young anorexic patients through family therapy. This method was developed by child psychiatrist Christopher Dare, psychologist Ivan Eisler and colleagues at the Institute of Psychiatry and Maudsley Hospital in London. Daniel La Grange, a clinical psychologist who is introducing the therapy at the University of Chicago, says, *The treatment is designed to empower the parents to take charge of their daughter's eating, to wrestle the eating disorder away from the adolescent so that the healthy adolescent has room to maneuver again* (Chicago Tribune, 1999). A study cited in the *Journal of the American Academy of Child and Adolescent Psychiatry* compared the effectiveness of family systems therapy with that of individual therapy. Both were found to be effective forms of treatment, but the behavioral systems therapy produced a faster return to health (Robin AL, 1999).

Another therapy looks at food sensitivities, especially among bulimics and binge eaters. Many people become addicted to the very foods they cannot tolerate. People can control their eating disorder more effectively by removing trigger foods, avoiding overly processed foods, and regulating blood sugar by eating proteins and fats with carbohydrates. Kay Sheppard outlines how to easily do this in her book, *From the First Bite: A Complete Guide to Recovery from Food Addiction* (Sheppard K, 2000).

OBESITY AS AN EATING DISORDER

One of the most common disorders affecting our children and adolescents today is obesity. Jeffrey P. Koplan, Director of the Center for Disease Control and Prevention, reported findings of a growing obesity epidemic in the United States spreading rapidly during the 1990s across all states, regions and demographic groups. The highest increase occurred among the youngest ages (18–29 years old), people with some college education and people of Hispanic ethnicity. Koplan cited the American lifestyle of convenience and inactivity as devastating to the health of children. Research shows that 60 percent of overweight 5 to 10-year-old children already have at least one risk factor for heart disease, including high cholesterol, elevated blood pressure and/or insulin levels (Mokdad AH, et. al., 1999).

How can I stop my child from obsessing about weight?

Although being overly concerned about body image at a young age can foster bulimia and anorexia, obesity among children is more pervasive. As a parent, the smartest way to deal with this delicate balance is to stress healthy eating instead of dieting. Most importantly, parents should "practice what they preach."

Making weight criticisms often makes the child more self-conscious and starts a pattern of yo-yo dieting. Instead of asking your child, *Are you sure you want that ice cream bar? Your stomach is protruding*, it would be far better to keep only healthy foods in your house so you don't have to be a "food cop." Also downplaying Hollywood's view of beauty, with plastic surgery and unnatural thinness as the norm, may allow your child to achieve a more realistic view of body weight and physical beauty.

What is Obesity?

Obesity is defined as an abnormal amount of fat on the body. The term is used when someone is 20–30 percent over the weight that is considered normal for their gender based on age and height. An accurate assessment of body fat is the body mass index. The body mass index of a person is their weight divided by their height, squared. This value is compared to normative data based on age, sex and race. A body mass index greater than the 95th percentile for age and sex is an acceptable definition of obesity (Schwartz MW, et. al., 1997).

WHAT HEALTH RISKS DOES OBESITY POSE FOR MY CHILD?

Obesity can influence a child's body in many ways. Doctors are finding accelerated bone growth and skeletal maturation and decreased levels of testosterone in severely obese boys. In girls, accelerated physical maturation may occur with early onset of menstrual cycles, no menstrual cycles, or abnormal bleeding between menstrual cycles. Obese girls are also at risk for polycystic ovaries, cholelithiasis (gall stones), increased respiratory illnesses (associated with obesity in toddlers under two years of age), and most alarmingly, hypertension, high cholesterol, and increased insulin levels (Schwartz MW, et. al., 1997). Hypertension and elevated cholesterol levels increase a child's risk of cardiovascular disease later in life. Increased levels of glucose can lead to Type II diabetes, a form of diabetes in which the body does not produce or properly use insulin. Insulin is an important hormone needed to convert sugar, starches and other foods into energy used for daily living. With obesity, the pancreas, where insulin is made, becomes overwhelmed with the increased demand for insulin. Continually overfeeding the body causes a resistance to insulin as well as an inability of the pancreas to produce it. Fewer than four percent of childhood diabetes cases in 1990 were Type II. That number has risen to approximately 20 percent, varying from 8 percent to 45 percent, depending upon the age of the group studied. Children who overeat, are sedentary, and have a family history of diabetes are at a higher risk for Type II diabetes (American Diabetes Association, March 2000). Doctors are especially concerned that prepubescent children who are getting less exercise, overeating nutritionally "empty" foods, and spending more time in front of televisions and computers may be increasing their risk for many health problems, Type II diabetes among them.

WHY IS THERE A SURGE IN OBESITY, ESPECIALLY AMONG CHILDREN?

At least one child in five is overweight in the United States. Over the last two decades this number has increased by more than 50 percent. The number of extremely overweight children has nearly doubled (Schwartz MW, et. al., 1997). While there are some types of obesity that are secondary to other diseases, these types account for only five percent of obesity in children. The remaining 95 percent of obese cases are attributed to excess caloric intake. Put another way, *obesity results from an excess of caloric intake over energy expenditure* (Center for Science in the Public Interest, January/February 2001). Factors that influence increased caloric intake in the United States are many while factors that influence increased daily physical activity are on the decline.

Yale University obesity expert, Kelly Brownell, feels that our food trends in the United States are part of the problem. *The promotion of high-fat and high-calorie foods goes on unabated. Food is more accessible and cheaper than ever* (Center for Science in the Public Interest, January/February 2001). Brownell cites toxic food environments as being the biggest culprit. Children have easy access to high-fat and high in calories food at almost every gas station, shopping mall, convenience store, vending machine, ballpark, movie theater, restaurant, and their own schools. Television advertisements, jingles, toys and celebrity endorsements encourage our children to eat junk food. Brownell also points out that we are expending fewer calories on physical activity than we used to as computers become a part of our everyday life and work (Center for Science in the Public Interest, January/February 2001).

Food addictions also play a role in overeating and obesity. Your child may be addicted to certain foods because of a food sensitivity or allergy (see Chapter 1 for details). The February 1992 edition of *The Nutrition and Dietary Consultant* describes how your child can become addicted to certain foods. *Physiologically, when a person (often a child) first has contact with an offending food, there is a response, usually unfavorable (headache, nausea, vomiting, gas, discomfort, asthma, congestion, rash, irritability, etc.). As the person continues to eat the food, the symptoms reduce and finally disappear. It is usually at this time that it is said that the child outgrows his allergies or stuffy nose, ear infections or upset stomach. In actuality, the food has now become habit and the symptoms are masked or delayed. The body has adapted to the offending substance and the body learns to live with it. However, there is a continuous stress on the system. In a confused effort to deal with the problem, the body now mistakes the offending substance for a nontoxic substance; and in the adaptation process the body actually becomes used to and dependent on the food. It is during this adaptation or masking phase that the addiction takes place. The physiological compensation of an allergy results in addiction and takes its toll in chronic stress. The adaptation is so strong that one becomes dependent or "hooked," eating the addictive food at regular intervals to avoid withdrawal symptoms. When you go without it for awhile or try to quit, your body craves the substance – the allergy/addiction syndrome. During the final stage, the body fails to maintain adaptation and experiences the allergic and addicted symptomatology simultaneously. During this stage, the chronic stage, the symptoms of chronic disease emerge. Scientists call this stage exhaustion and during exhaustion the allergy resurfaces in full force* (Reno EG, 1992).

HOW IS OBESITY TREATED?

In obesity, there is an imbalance in energy intake and expenditure. If put on a low calorie diet, an obese person's ability to burn calories actually decreases. Therefore, simply putting your child on a reduced-calorie diet may exacerbate the problem. A successful treatment plan should include testing for food allergies and determining whether there are food addictions. Prevention is ultimately the best way of avoiding obesity. Since statistics show that 25 percent of obese infants and 50 percent of adolescent girls remain obese into adulthood, it is important to take a proactive role in your child's life. Encourage physical activity and strive to make it an important part of every day. Teach your child to make food and lifestyle choices that are healthful. Support your community's physical education programs and proactively encourage your policymakers to provide recreational areas and to offer healthy food choices in your child's school cafeteria (Mokdad AH, et. al., 1999).

Personal Case Study #8

Judy was probably my most challenging client early in my career. She was a 22-year-old bulimic who was obese and emotionally scarred. She had tried several times to commit suicide ever since age 13 and had just been released from her third in-patient eating disorders clinic where she was force-fed and purged each time. Her mother said that I was her last hope.

Through previous food sensitivity tests, Judy had shown reactions to her favorite foods (corn products, wheat, yeast, and cow's milk products). She couldn't control her intake when she began eating any of these foods, but felt so bloated and nauseated several hours later that she purged, as she described, *in the way a person vomits when they have the flu.*

She was very deficient in all B-vitamins, zinc, magnesium, calcium, and protein. For two weeks, I supplemented her with these and other nutrients. She was instructed to eat protein foods at each meal. I also gave her acidophilus and digestive enzymes to resolve her grossly impaired digestion.

The third week, when she felt ready, we removed all of her "trigger" foods at once. I gave her satisfying substitutes for her favorites. That week was very difficult. She felt exhausted, headachy, and achy all over. On the tenth day after withdrawal, she said, "I have a feeling of energy more powerful than I knew was possible. I knew then that I had turned the corner." She lost 12 pounds of fluid in two weeks.

Judy is now a 35-year-old mother of two who works part-time as a therapist. She counsels teenagers and young women who suffer from eating disorders. She is proud of the fact that she hasn't had a binge or purge in 13 years!

Dr. Holk's RX

Obesity is on the rise in both adults and children. This is of special concern because obesity is a preventable condition. Overweight children often become overweight adults and overweight adults are at higher risk for many serious health problems including: heart disease, high blood pressure, stroke, high cholesterol, diabetes, some cancers, and depression.

Since most children learn their eating habits by watching those around them, it is important for the family to play an active role in the lifestyle and dietary modifications that have to be made to insure gradual and permanent change. It is a myth that children can eat anything and remain healthy. Children need to be educated about proper nutrition and its role in the maintenance of health. As a parent, it is important for you to be a role model. Evaluate your own eating habits. See if you can identify where you are displaying an unwanted behavior that your child may be mimicking. It may be necessary to change your nutritional habits or exercise routine before asking your child to do the same. In doing so you act as a positive role model for your child.

To help your child, focus on healthy eating and increasing physical activity for the whole family. Below are some ideas to help you get started.

- Plan time for family excursions that involve physical activity.
- Incorporate exercise into your daily routine.
- Plan to have the family eat nutritious meals together at a set time each day.

- Eat slowly so that the body's signals of satiety can be recognized (it takes 15 minutes for the brain to tell your stomach that it is full).
- Choose to eat nutritionally dense foods.
- Help your child to distinguish between hunger and craving (unless your child's stomach is growling, your child is not truly hungry).
- Allow your child to become involved in food selection and preparation.
- Discourage eating or snacking while watching TV or working on the computer.
- Discourage skipping meals.
- Offer nutritious options for snacks.
- Do not use food as a reward – a hug works much better!

Children who are overweight often suffer from depression and low self-esteem. Therefore, it is imperative to recognize your children's emotional needs. Love and support them unconditionally without passing judgement or blaming them for *their* problem. As previously stated, a child's eating habits often mimic the habits of those around them. It is important that the whole family make lifestyle and dietary changes.

Seek other professionals such as doctors, nutritionists, and psychologists for support. Be willing to take your child to a doctor for evaluation to rule out any metabolic pathologies that may be present. Common blood tests can be used to generally evaluate the status of electrolytes, proteins, the blood, the liver, the thyroid gland, and the kidneys. This information will give clues as to the imbalances that need to be corrected. A restrictive type of diet, especially with a child under the age of two, should be supervised by a qualified health care professional. Restrictive diets may interfere with your child's development.

Allergies and food cravings are important to identify and address. Allergies are a warning sign that foods may be creating an imbalance. Removing common offenders (milk, cheese, wheat, corn, etc.) from the diet often helps to eliminate the allergies. Children often crave the food to which they most react.

I have also found the use of homeopathy to be very helpful in working with the physical, emotional, and mental aspects of eating disorders. Homeopathy in conjunction with professional counseling can be very effective. To find a homeopathic practitioner in you area, contact one of the following organizations.

American Institute of Homeopathy
801 N. Fairfax Street, Suite 306
Alexandria, Virginia 22314
Phone: (888) 445-9988
Website: *www.homeopathyusa.org*

Council for Homeopathic Certification
1060 North 4th Street
San Jose, CA 95112
Phone: (408) 971-5915

Homeopathic Academy of Naturopathic Physicians
12132 S.E. Foster Place
Portland, OR 97266
Phone: (503) 761-3298
Website: *www.healthy.net/hanp*

North American Society of Homeopaths
1122 East Pike Street, # 1122
Seattle, WA 98122
Phone: (206) 720-7000
Website: *www.homeopathy.org*

﹎❨ 9 ❩﹏

Depression and Violence

The teenage years are difficult and, according to Jean M. Twenge, Ph.D., filled with more anxiety today than they were thirty years ago. The average American child in the 1980s reported more anxiety than child psychiatric patients in the 1950s (Twenge, 2000). Dr. Twenge's research suggests that one's level of anxiety is directly correlated to one's sense of social connectedness and inversely correlated with one's perception of environmental danger. In other words, a strong sense of belonging and social connectedness is associated with a lesser degree of anxiety; a strong sense of environmental danger such as violent crime, is associated with a higher level of anxiety. She commented that *until people feel both safe and connected to others, anxiety is likely to remain high* (Twenge, 2000).

It is estimated that up to 2.5 percent of children and up to 8.3 percent of adolescents in the U.S. suffer from depression in one of its many forms (Birmaher, et. al., 1996). Depression has been found to be associated with poor scholastic performance, fear of school, eating disorders, panic attacks, increased anxiety, delinquency, and other conduct disorders (Weinberg, et. al., 1995). It is also the leading cause of suicide. Weinberg, et. al. state that *Death wishes occur in 35 percent of prepubertal children manifesting depression, suicidal ideation (thoughts and plans) in 15 percent, and suicidal attempts in 5 percent* (Weinberg, et. al., 1995).

Depressive disorders are not well recognized in the young population because of the variability with which the symptoms may present. Parents are quick to accept that adolescence is a time of moodiness and defiance and so are hesitant to label their child as depressed or to seek medical help to address their concerns. Medical personal may also be hesitant to assign a diagnosis of depression to a child recognizing the stigma that often accompanies the diagnosis of mental illness. Yet, early detection and treatment of depression is imperative for your child's emotional, physical and social well being.

WHAT DO I LOOK FOR IF I SUSPECT MY CHILD IS DEPRESSED?

When five or more of the following symptoms persist in children, adolescents, or adults for two or more weeks, a diagnosis of depression is appropriate.

- Persistent sad or irritable mood
- Loss of interest in activities once enjoyed
- Significant change in appetite or body weight
- Difficulty sleeping or oversleeping
- Psychomotor agitation or retardation
- Loss of energy
- Feelings of worthlessness or inappropriate guilt
- Difficulty concentrating
- Recurrent thoughts of death or suicide

Source: American Psychiatric Association. *Diagnostic and Statistical Manual of Mental Disorders*, 4th ed. (DSM-IV). Washington DC: American Psychiatric Press, 1994.

Since depression in children and adolescents may take on many forms, ranging from complete withdraw to violent aggression, the following signs may also be present:

- Frequent, vague, non-specific physical complaints such as headaches, muscle aches, stomachaches, or fatigue
- Frequent absences from school or poor performance in school
- Talk of or efforts to run away from home
- Outbursts of shouting, complaining, unexplained irritability, or crying
- Lack of interest in playing with friends

- Alcohol or substance abuse
- Social isolation, poor communication
- Fear of death
- Extreme sensitivity to rejection or failure
- Inability to accept compliments, rewards or awards
- Increased irritability, anger, or hostility
- Reckless behavior
- Difficulty with relationships
- Excessive fighting, hostility, belligerence
- Lack of respect for authority

RISK FACTORS FOR DEPRESSION

In adolescence, girls are twice as likely as boys to develop depression. In childhood, girls and boys are at equal risk (Birmaher, et. al., 1996). A family history of the disorder is positively correlated with depression in children and adolescents, but the correlation is not as strong with adolescents. Depressed children who are oppositional and defiant or who have another conduct disorder often have a positive family history for alcoholism (Weinberg, et. al, 1995). The National Institute of Mental Health (NIMH), part of the National Institutes of Health (NIH), identifies the following additional risk factors (NIMH, 2001).

- Stress
- Cigarette smoking
- A loss of a parent or loved one
- Attentional, conduct or learning disorders
- Chronic illnesses, such as diabetes
- Abuse or neglect
- Other trauma, including natural disasters

WHAT CAN I DO TO HELP MY CHILD'S MENTAL HEALTH?

Although more studies are needed, data is beginning to show that children who have poor communication and less intimacy with their parents are more prone to disruptive behavior, low academic achievement, depression, and substance abuse (Silver, 2000). In recognition of this, experts are emphasizing the important role parents play in the mental health of their children and are promoting open communication between parents and children. A study published in *Psychology of Addictive Behaviors* cited the important role mother-teen communication played in influencing a teen's choice about binge-drinking. The authors stated they were *impressed with the consistency with which mother-teen communications influenced the 'beliefs' that prevented the experience of negative consequences associated with binge-drinking* (Turrisi, et. al., 2001).

Encourage your child to share their thoughts and feelings. Listen attentively and without judgement. Acknowledge their feelings as being valid and offer hope, when possible, without belittling their concerns. Recognize that talk of suicide should be taken seriously and a professional healthcare provider should be consulted. Talk with your children honestly about your love and concern for them and be assured that what you say and do will make a difference in their lives.

TEEN VIOLENCE

Teen violence is often associated with depression. A recent study in the *Journal of the American Academy of Child and Adolescent Psychiatry* cited that of the depressed teens identified for the study, *70 percent reported a history of 'frequent' verbal aggression at home, 24 percent reported frequent physical aggression in the home, 30 percent reported receiving detentions at school for aggression, and 14 percent reported being arrested for aggressive behavior* (Knox, et. al, 2000). The reason for the association between violence and depression has not been found but an abnormal level of serotonin, a brain neurotransmitter, is suspect.

Another issue that cannot be ignored is heavy metal toxicity through constant exposure from birth to copper, mercury, lead, cadmium, and arsenic. William Walsh, Ph.D., of the Pfeiffer Treatment Center, has proven an association between heavy metal toxicity and mass murders (Walsh, Nolta News, 2000).

DATE VIOLENCE

A recent shocking study by the Harvard School of Public Health discovered that one in five high school girls reports being a victim of physical or sexual violence in a dating relationship (Silverman, August, 2001). One of the most disturbing aspects of dating violence is that teen girls who experience it tend to adopt risky behaviors. For instance, victimized girls were:

- 8–9 times more likely to attempt suicide
- 4–6 times more likely to have used cocaine, and
- 3–4 times more likely to have used unhealthy dieting methods such as vomiting and laxatives.

Although violence against women is a major public health issue, there are few services in place for victims of dating violence. One of the reasons for this is that 65 percent of the abused teen girls did not tell anyone.

Teen boys learn violence toward women from family or cultural behaviors. Interventions must begin with parents and schools teaching kids **before** dating age that all violence is unacceptable and that demanding and giving respect in all peer relationships is mandatory. Teen girls and their parents need to know the warning signs of an abusive relationship. Having a jealous boyfriend or one who tries to control his girlfriend's appearance may seem romantic but these behaviors are not healthy. Parent and teacher discussions of date violence, support groups initiated by high school counselors, and questions asked by pediatricians can give victims of this hidden epidemic a chance to heal their pain and humiliation.

THERAPIES TO TREAT DEPRESSION

Treatment for depression and conduct disorders often includes a combination of psychotherapy, medication, and environmental modifications at home and in school. Many different forms of psychotherapy are available. Cognitive-behavioral therapy (CBT) and interpersonal therapy (IPT) are two forms recommended by the National Institute of Mental Health (NIMH) as being effective for children and adolescents.

The effectiveness of antidepressant medications for children and adolescents has not yet been thoroughly researched. Antidepressant medication can be an effective form of therapy for adults when used in conjunction with psychotherapy, but the same is not known to be true for children and adolescents. According to the National Institute of Mental Health, there are only two controlled studies that support the efficacy of floxetine (Prosac®) and paroxetine (Paxil®). No research has supported the use of tricyclic antidepressants for children.

Even though medications may effectively treat depression among children and teens, concern has been mounting over their side-effects. Prozac® was first made available in 1986 and is now the world's most widely prescribed antidepressant with more than 38 million people using it worldwide. Severe side-effects have been cited. A study, published by Dr. David Healy in *Primary Care Psychiatry*, found that two out of twenty healthy volunteers who were put on Prozac® became suicidal compared to none in the control group who were on a different antidepressant. As a parent, make sure you fully understand the possible side-effects of any medication prescribed for your child, and educate yourself about signs and symptoms that may be a warning of possible danger.

The Physician's Desk Reference lists the following as possible side effects for fluoxetine hydrochloride (Prozac®).

- Gastrointestinal disturbances, dyspepsia, abdominal pain, diarrhea

- Anorexia and weight loss
- Headache
- Nervousness, anxiety, dizziness, tremor
- Dry mouth
- Convulsions
- Fever
- Sexual dysfunction
- Sweating
- Blood sugar changes with increased sugar cravings
- Confusion, drowsiness
- Hypertension
- Palpitations
- Asthenia (lack or loss of strength usually of muscular or cerebellar origin)
- Movement disorders and dyskinesias (defect in voluntary movement)
- Neuroleptic malignant syndrome type event (The combination of catatonic rigidity, stupor, unstable blood pressure, hyperthermia, profuse sweating, air hunger, and incontinence that occurs as a toxic reaction to use of potent antipsychotic agents in therapeutic doses. These may last five to ten days after discontinuation of the drug) (Thomas CL, ed., 1989).
- Cerebral vascular accident (stroke)
- Hypomania
- Manic reactions
- Delusions, psychosis, paranoia
- Suicidal ideation
- Violent behavior, hostility

Physician's Desk Reference, 2000, pp. 962-966.

Given that hostility, paranoia, delusions, psychosis, and manic reactions are considered to be infrequent but potentially real side effects of Prozac®, it is possible that the use of Prozac® and similar drugs may be contributing to the increase in violence (murders, suicides, road rage, etc.). We know that Eric Harris, the teenage gunman in the Columbine High School shootings, was taking a prescribed antidepressant drug.

While sitting on the patio of my La Jolla home to write this chapter, I was interrupted by my husband shouting that a high school student had opened fire in his San Diego suburban high school. At least one student was known dead. When will this kind of psychotic behavior end? I know when I was in high school, these kinds of episodes never occurred, not even in the most dangerous ghettos in Chicago.

ARE THERE NATURAL METHODS FOR HELPING VIOLENT OR DEPRESSED YOUTH?

Diet and exercise play important roles in overall health and vitality and are considered essential when working with someone who suffers from depression or violence. Studies have demonstrated the efficacy of nutritional supplementation and the removal of sugar and chemical additives from the diets of emotionally challenged youngsters. Botanicals such as St John's Wort and *Vitex agnus cactus* may be helpful. Environmental allergies, nutritional deficiencies, food sensitivities, and heavy metal toxicity should also be ruled out.

When I counsel a child or teenager who is violent or depressed, I take the following steps:

1. I make sure they are receiving appropriate mental health therapy.

2. I require the results of a blood test to rule out or identify anemia, mineral deficiencies, blood sugar imbalance, liver impairment, allergies, etc.

3. If necessary, I request urine, hair, and/or blood analysis to rule out heavy metal toxicity or drug abuse. William Walsh, Ph.D., director of the Pfeiffer Treatment Center, has identified zinc/copper imbalance as a major offender in many mass murders. He also identified an experimental drug intended to treat depression as the culprit in at least one mass murder.

4. I recommend dietary supplementation of a multi-vitamin and mineral containing a substantial amount of B-vitamins. I always add magnesium because it is the most deficient nutrient among most depressed or violent kids. As needed, I'll add zinc, calcium, iron, and/or digestive enzymes.

5. I recommend a diet that is nutrient-dense with adequate protein and healthy fats. I recommend restricting or avoiding all sugar, soft drinks, artificial colors, and most sugar substitutes.

6. If food sensitivities are suspected, I recommend a two-week Elimination Diet (see Chapter 13 for details) to determine the offending food(s).

7. If food or environmental allergies are suspected, I refer to an allergist for further testing.

I have been dismayed to find that **none** of the violent or depressed youth I have counseled were given blood tests by their psychiatrist to rule out organic nutritional imbalances before being prescribed medication. Yet, every one of these youngsters displayed at least one major nutritional imbalance. The best way parents can ensure appropriate mental health care for their children is to insist on blood and urine testing before medicating.

Personal Case Study #9

John was a violent, depressed seventeen-year-old teenager when he walked into my office. His mother decided to send him alone because he was so cruel to her that he would scream insults at her and punch his fist through walls when something irked him. He was huge (6'2", 245 pounds) and had a severe case of acne. His mother told me he had no friends (other students were afraid of his volatile behavior) and that his grades were mostly Ds and Fs.

John would not sit down at our first session. He paced the room for the first few minutes. He then said, *Lady, if you think I'm going to give up drinking milk, I am leaving right now* (his mother had warned him that I said people are usually reactive to foods they crave). I asked John how much milk he drank. He said, *I drink at least a gallon of milk and eat a gallon of ice cream every day.* When I asked him what other foods he ate daily, he shot back, *Not much.*

John clearly had a milk allergy, later diagnosed by an allergist. His blood calcium level was also the lowest the allergist had ever seen. John craved milk products because he was calcium deficient, but he couldn't absorb them due to his cow's milk allergy. It is a known fact that severe calcium, magnesium, and zinc deficiencies can cause violent behavior.

It took John three months before his supplements of calcium, magnesium, and Vitamin D stopped his milk craving. After six months, he began losing weight, his acne disappeared, his grades skyrocketed, and he became a pleasant young man. At his present age of twenty-five, he has become a police officer and the community's designated "Officer Friendly." He routinely tells me that he's licked his addiction and has been milk-free for seven years.

DR. HOLK'S RX: ST. JOHN'S WORT

This herb has been well researched in the other countries, and its use for the treatment of depression is widely accepted. There have not been many studies done with children so it is imperative to work with a health care practitioner when considering the use of any herb for children. Dosages vary according to age, weight, and other variables. Herbs can potentiate the action of other drugs, which may lead to life-threatening consequences. The consumption of certain foods may also be contraindicated. The information below is to be used as a guideline and is not meant to take the place of your health care practitioner's advice. See your health care practitioner before using any herb for medicinal purposes.

ST. JOHN'S WORT (HYPERICUM PERFORATUM)

St. John's wort is listed in the *Physicians' Desk Reference (PDR) for Herbal Medicines* as having mild antidepressant, sedative, and anti-anxiety properties (PDR, 1998). The use of St. John's wort as a natural antidepressant has been thoroughly researched. Studies show the herb inhibits the uptake of serotonin and acts like other selective serotonin reuptake inhibitors (Prozac®, Paxal®, Zoloft®, etc.) but with less cost and fewer side effects. St. John's wort can be used in cases of depression, anxiety, insomnia, apathy, and sleep disturbance (Pizzorno, 2000).

Caution should be used in combining prescription selective serotonin reuptake inhibitors (SSRI's) or monoamine oxidase inhibitors (MAO's) with St. John's Wort due to the possibility of potentiating the effect of these drugs (Holzl J, Demisch L, Gollnik B., 1989; Okpanyi SN, Weischer ML., 1987; McGuffin M, Hobbs C, Upton R, Goldberg A., 1997; Brown R., 1997; Rasmussen P., 1998). The use of St. John's wort is contraindicated in pregnancy and while taking narcotics and over-the-counter cold and flu medications. Do not use this herb while consuming alcohol or with those who are on drugs that stimulate the sympathetic nervous system (asthmatics). Avoid tyramine-containing foods such as pickled herring, cheeses, wine, beer, bananas, soft drinks, pineapples, yogurt, chocolate, peanuts and pastrami (Ronzio RA, 1997).

SECTION TWO

WHAT WE CAN DO TO HELP THEM

❦ 10 ❦

Start at the Very Beginning to Ensure Optimum Health for your Child

HOW TO OPTIMIZE YOUR CHILD'S HEALTH BEFORE CONCEPTION:

Six months before planned conception is the minimum time necessary to remove caffeine, overly processed foods, additives such as aspartame, food dyes, and monosodium glutamate, and alcohol from your diet. If you smoke cigarettes, or take even an occasional over-the-counter medication or recreational drug, discontinue them. If you are taking a prescription drug or herbal treatment for a medical condition, discuss with your obstetrician or family practitioner its safety during pregnancy. For instance, anti-seizure drugs and anti-depressants taken during pregnancy account for higher than normal incidents of birth defects among babies. If your medication may be unsafe during pregnancy, your physician will either discontinue your medication or switch you to an alternative.

Minimize your exposure to environmental, workplace, and household toxins (see Chapter 11 for more details).

Three months before planned conception is the minimum time necessary to remove excess simple sugar carbohydrates and any allergenic or reactive foods from your diet. Eat three balanced meals that contain protein and healthy fats at each meal. If you snack, choose nutrient-dense items such as nuts/seeds with fruit or guacamole with raw vegetables.

At intended conception, eat more alkaline and less acidic foods. See Chapter 14 for further details. Excess acid in your body can kill sperm. Also, limit exposure to high estrogen items such as soy, some cow's milk products, chlorinated water, ginseng, dong quai, and coffee.

141

Too much estrogen with too little progesterone may make it more difficult to conceive or may cause miscarriage.

Is my prenatal supplement enough?

All prenatal supplements today contain adequate amounts of folic acid (800-1000 mcg.). Most, however, do not contain enough magnesium to prevent the common complaints and health risks of pregnancy and delivery. I recommend 300-500 mg. of highly absorbable magnesium to all of my clients who are planning pregnancies. Adding extra vitamin B_6 to your prenatal supplement will encourage optimum immune system, brain, and behavior development of the fetus, may prevent miscarriage, and can minimize morning sickness

Many research studies have shown that extra vitamin C (usually 500 mg.) and zinc (20–30 mg.) taken by both the mother and father before and at conception may prevent subtle birth defects and allow sperm to "swim" faster. Most prenatal supplements do not contain enough vitamin C. Be sure to take a zinc-containing supplement after a protein meal (preferably after lunch or dinner) to prevent nausea.

My main complaint with most prescribed prenatal supplements is that they contain too much iron (some have 90 mg.) which is constipating, fights zinc absorption, and is not necessary the first trimester. The ferric form, which is in most inexpensive prenatals, is not well absorbed at any time. (The ferrous form is to be preferred.) When women are already feeling queasy the first trimester, too much iron makes them feel much worse (adequate daily iron intake for most females during the first trimester of pregnancy is 18–36 mg.).

I recommend that prenatal supplements be taken after a lunch or dinner protein meal. Many pregnant women stop taking their prenatal supplements due to adverse effects. Some women react adversely to prenatal supplements due to food sensitivities. If you react to your prenatal supplement for whatever reason, or it contains too much iron, it may be best to find a more acceptable one or to avoid a prenatal and take individual vitamins and minerals; including a low dose of B-complex, extra folic acid, magnesium, zinc, iron (in the ferrous form), and calcium to meet the demands of pregnancy. It is important to work with a knowledgeable health professional in planning the appropriate prenatal supplements.

WHEN I AM PREGNANT, SHOULD I EAT DIFFERENTLY THAN PRE-CONCEPTION?

The main difference in food intake from an optimum pre-conception diet to a pregnancy diet is to add more protein, carbohydrates, and fats to meet the growth needs of the fetus. Also, be careful to avoid most herbal teas (they can be allergenic and can block iron absorption), avoid eating high-in-mercury fish (see Table I: Fish Advisory), avoid all raw animal products (including sushi), avoid peanut-containing items completely (peanut is the most life threatening allergen of children), and increase dietary and supplemental calcium during the second and third trimesters to reach a level of 1200 mg. daily. Magnesium intake should be at least 500 mg. (from supplements and food). If you get any muscle cramps in your legs or feet, increase magnesium intake by 100 mg. increments until the cramping stops.

TABLE I: FDA FISH HEALTH ADVISORY FOR PREGNANT/LACTATING WOMEN (to avoid mercury toxicity)

Fish to Avoid	Fish intake of 12 oz. maximum weekly
tuna steaks	canned tuna
oysters (Gulf of Mexico)	mahi mahi
marlin	blue mussels
halibut	eastern oyster
pike	cod
walleye	pollack
white croaker	salmon from Great Lakes
largemouth bass	blue crab (Gulf of Mexico)
all raw fish	

Source: *Food and Drug Administration Health Advisory, 2001*

WHAT CAN I DO FOR MORNING SICKNESS?

"Morning sickness" is the dated term for the nausea and vomiting (NVP) of pregnancy. Many studies have shown that NVP during the first trimester of pregnancy actually indicates a healthy pregnancy and less incidence of miscarriage.

Women who have a history of nausea and vomiting after estrogen exposure, a history of motion sickness, or who have an acute sense of taste are the most likely to experience NVP, according to Murphy Goodwin, M.D., Chief of the Maternal-Fetal Medicine Department of the Women and Children's Hospital in Los Angeles (*Nutrition and the M.D.*, June 2001). If NVP begins after ten weeks, if the vomiting is associated with maternal weight loss, or if NVP interferes with a woman's activities and responsibilities of daily life, it needs to be addressed by your physician. If other causes of NVP have been ruled out, the following therapies have been shown to reduce or eliminate NVP entirely:

- High protein meals (the high carbohydrate, low fat recommendations of the past are ineffective and may worsen or prolong NVP);
- Addition of Vitamin B_6 to the prenatal supplement (10–50 mg. daily);
- Ginger (in pill, tea, or chewed raw forms);
- Acupuncture/acupressure (including acupressure wrist bands);
- Eating small meals every few hours (always including protein, but may also include salty items such as salted nuts, pretzels, or saltine crackers to neutralize excess acid and to stimulate the adrenal glands).

If all of the above are ineffective, one of the following may be necessary:

- Physician-prescribed B_6 plus doxylamine
- Physician-ordered intravenous hydration

(**Primary Source:** Goodwin. *Nutrition & the M.D.*, Vol. 27, No. 6, June 2001.)

I'M A VEGETARIAN. CAN I STILL HAVE A HEALTHY PREGNANCY?

Women who are deficient in Vitamin B_{12} may be at risk for infertility or repeated miscarriages, according to recent studies reported in the *Journal of Reproductive Medicine* (JRM 2001; 46:209-212). Vitamin B_{12} plays a key role in promoting a healthy nervous system, development of new tissue, and ovulation. If women are deficient in B_{12}, which is found only in animal foods unless supplemented, a fertilized egg may not develop, resulting in miscarriage. If sufficient B_{12} in supplement form (I usually recommend 100–200 mcg. for vegetarian clients) or through injection is given, this situation can usually be reversed.

In my experience, adding more protein from compatible animal sources will increase chances of fertility, less miscarriages, and healthier pregnancies. As an intern at the March of Dimes Birth Defects Foundation thirteen years ago, I noticed that most pregnant vegetarians did not consume enough protein during pregnancy. They had many pregnancy and birth complications directly related to lack of B_{12} and protein. Today, I recommend, in addition to an excellent prenatal supplement with extra B_6 and B_{12}, the following to all of my vegetarian clients:

- If vegan, I convince them to add organic eggs and/or dairy products to their diet during pregnancy to reach the recommended 70–80 grams of daily protein needed to achieve an **optimum** pregnancy.
- If they are eating more than 10 grams of soy protein daily (including soy protein powder), I switch them to organic whey protein powder (unless they are dairy allergic).
- I add at least one-half cup of raw or dry roasted nuts/seeds (except peanuts) to their daily food intake to provide healthy fat and an extra protein source.
- If they are willing to eat fish, I recommend at least 6 oz. of safe fish sources every other day.

**WHAT, BESIDES EATING WELL AND TAKING MY SUPPLEMENTS, WILL
HELP ME ACHIEVE A HEALTHY PREGNANCY AND DELIVERY?**

It is not within the scope of this book to give detailed
explanations of medical procedures. That should be the
role of a licensed health practitioner in charge of your
prenatal care. However, the March of Dimes Birth Defects
Foundation, double-blind research studies, and experts in
the field of maternal-fetal medicine encourage the following considerations to optimize the health of you and your
child:

- Begin professional prenatal care within the first
  trimester of pregnancy and continue until six weeks
  postpartum.

- Avoid too little or too much weight gain during
  pregnancy (the U.S. Institute of Medicine recommends an ideal weight gain of 25–35 pounds for
  women whose pre-pregnancy weight was normal).

- Test for gestational diabetes, anemia, and other
  pregnancy related health risks at appropriate times
  during pregnancy. If health risks are discovered,
  they need to be dealt with immediately by your
  prenatal specialist.

- Avoid unnecessary pregnancy and birth interventions. Research has found that ultrasound, electronic
  fetal monitoring, routine episiotomies, forceps deliveries, medications, especially to stimulate labor, and
  cesarean deliveries are overused and often contraindicated. For example, although rates of cesarean
  delivery dropped from 1989–1996, they are rising
  again (up to 22 percent in 1999). One of the reasons
  for this rise in cesarean deliveries is an alarming
  trend by some obstetricians to encourage cesareans
  upon demand for **nonmedical** reasons. Even the
  American College of Obstetricians and Gynecologists
  president, W. Benson Harer, Jr., M.D., recommends
  that the mother's choice be the deciding factor for a
  cesarean delivery (*Nat'l. Women's Health Network*

News, July/August 2001). If your obstetrician recommends cesarean delivery upon demand, this is a "red flag" for potentially unsafe obstetrical management.

- For low risk pregnancies and the most natural childbirth preferences, consider using a midwife or doula during your pregnancy and delivery and/or a physician-attended homebirth. Most individuals who opt for these "out-of-the-norm" birthing situations are conscientious college graduates who have scientifically researched the pros and cons of a wide variety of birthing situations and have decided that the more natural the birth, the happier the mother and the healthier the infant. For more information regarding natural birthing, contact the American College of Nurse Midwives (*www.midwife.org*; 202-728-9860), Doulas of North America (*www.dona.org*; 801-756-7331), Midwives Alliance of North America (*www.mana.org*; 316-283-4543), and Homefirst Health Services (*www.homefirst.com*, 847-679-8336).

- Avoid unnecessary risks during pregnancy. Leave the jogging, skiing, and hang-gliding for another time (even if you are an expert in these sports). Always wear a seat belt and avoid flying in an airplane during the last four-six weeks of pregnancy (or as directed by your licensed health professional).

- Exercise safely. Avoid putting pressure on the abdominal area with heavy lifting, sit-ups, etc.

- Enjoy pregnancy. It may be one of the few times in your life that you will be consistently pampered and adored. You don't even have to worry about your figure. Remember that pregnancy and childbirth are normal, healthy processes. The awesome power and responsibility of bringing another healthy and productive human being into the world due to your nurturing and love (in utero and out) should be one of your proudest and most joyful moments.

BREAST IS BEST

Oliver Wendel Holmes once said, "Breasts are more skillful at compounding a feeding mixture than the hemispheres of the most learned professor's brain" (Eisenstein, *Safer Medicine*, 2000, p. 91). There is clear evidence that a breast-fed baby, especially in the first six months of life, has dramatic lifelong advantages over bottle-fed infants. Some of these advantages include fewer cases of:

- Allergy
- Eczema
- Asthma
- Ear infections
- Bronchitis
- Pneumonia
- Diarrhea
- Constipation

The immune and digestive systems of breastfed infants become stronger than bottle-fed infants, especially if the mother eats an optimum, allergy-free diet while nursing. I usually recommend a diet similar to the prenatal diet, continuation of the prenatal supplements, and avoidance of any food to which the mother or father has a known sensitivity.

Breast-feeding also enhances a child's intelligence. Because infants have brains and nervous systems that are growing at a rapid rate, the appropriate raw materials are required. Breast milk has them all.

I always recommend that nursing women avoid peanut protein because it has become such a life-threatening allergen for children. Several studies suggest that transfer of maternal dietary peanut protein to breast milk may predispose at risk children to acute sensitization (Ewan, *British Medical Journal*, 1996; 312:1074-8). Peanut allergy is the most common food-related cause of death among children.

I also counsel parents to avoid giving their child "peanut-containing" foods (including peanut butter) until their child is at least two years old (some pediatricians recommended not before age four) because of its allergy potential, and because the aflatoxin mold contained in most peanuts cannot be eradicated effectively by a young child's still-developing immune system.

IS THERE ANY INFANT FORMULA I CAN USE IF I CAN'T NURSE MY INFANT?

Nursing has been a very natural instinctive process of all mammals since the beginning of time. If a mother is having trouble breastfeeding, excellent sources for assistance can come from a parent or friend who nursed successfully, a lactation consultant, or a member of the LaLeche League. Infant formulas are not a magic concoction and no one, to date, has been able to bring it even close to the benefits of mother's milk. Cow's milk formulas, perfect for calves, but not humans, have been implicated in insulin-dependent juvenile diabetes, chronic diarrhea or constipation, ear infections, respiratory problems, viral infections, and eczema. Switching to soy formulas may improve some of the cow's milk symptoms, but pose unanswered questions of risks showing up in adulthood. In August 2001,the *Journal of the American Medical Association (JAMA)* called soy-based infant formulas safe for infants. After many months of speculation concerning the estrogen-like compounds (known as phytoestrogens) naturally present in soy posing a risk to developing infants, this was proved untrue by a long-term study of over eight hundred men and women who were fed a soy-based formula during infancy.

The most depressing, and completely irreversible problem of baby formulas in the U.S., is their lack of added essential fatty acids (EFAs). Formulas containing essential fatty acids have been used for years in Europe because they have been shown to exert a powerful influence on the developing brain membranes, which affect communication of brain cells. Intelligent Quotients (I.Q.s) of infants fed formulas containing essential fatty acids have been shown to increase by 10–15 percent. Because newborns can't manufacture all of the essential fats needed for optimal cognitive and visual development, a formula supplemented with these fats can improve a baby's eyesight. Many neurodevelopmental disorders that manifest in childhood, including Attention Deficit Disorder, dyslexia, and the autism spectrum can be minimized or prevented through the addition of essential fatty acids in infant formulas; which by the way, are found naturally in mother's milk (Richardson, *PLEFA* 2000; 63:1-9). The Child Health Foundation of Munich now recommends that all infant formulas be fortified with EFAs. After pressure was exerted by worldwide studies and by scientific experts, the FDA agreed in May 2001 to allow the addition of essential fatty acids, including DHA and AA fats, to infant formulas.

If my clients will not or cannot nurse, I often recommend the following:

- Choosing a formula that shows no overt physical reactions (constipation, diarrhea, projectile vomiting, eczema, chronic ear infections, etc.);
- Supplementing with essential fatty acids, such as cod liver oil and organic safflower or sunflower oil, if the infant formula does not already contain them;
- Choosing a formula that contains a natural source of lauric acid such as coconut oil (lauric acid is found naturally in mother's milk and is essential for strengthening an infant's immune system);
- Adding small doses of B-vitamins, zinc, and magnesium to the infant formula, dependent on age and weight, to optimize neurotransmission in the infant's brain;
- Adding probiotics (acidophilus with bifidus) in small doses to strengthen the infant's immune system and digestive tract. A recent study in Lancet showed resistance to allergic reactions and eczema in high-risk infants who were given probiotics. Another study showed an 80 percent lowered risk of develop-

ing diarrhea when hospitalized infants were given probiotics (*Journal of Pediatrics*, 2001; 138: 361-5).

The low rate of breast-feeding in the United States, especially among minorities, warrants action. The U.S. Department of Health and Human Services and American Academy of Pediatricians have become pro-active with public health announcements and brochures urging women to breastfeed for a full year. My words of encouragement to my clients who find breastfeeding inconvenient or problematical are: *Think of how quickly six months to a year passes by. If you can minimize or avoid doctor visits, antibiotics, behavioral problems, digestive distress, and learning issues for your breastfed children, you will have saved years of aggravation, worry, stress, wasted time, and lost money. The reward of growing happy, healthy children is well worth it!*

What can I do about the "baby blues"?

Postpartum depression, often referred to as the baby blues, is a common problem after childbirth. Statistics show that 80 percent of new mothers experience the problem to some degree. One in ten develops full-blown depression and one in a thousand develops postpartum psychosis. Believing that childbirth is a miraculous experience should not mean denying that it can be a physical, mental, and emotional strain for the mother. Psychiatric care, including the use of prescription anti-depressants, is often not the answer. Too little magnesium depleted in pregnancy, delivery, and postpartum along with hormonal imbalance after delivery often are at the root of postpartum depression.

If you even have a hint that you or a loved one might be suffering from postpartum depression, discuss options with a qualified healthcare practitioner. Some obstetricians have witnessed postpartum depression lifting in a few hours from a single injection of progesterone. Postpartum depression should never be trivialized or ignored. Too many mothers and children have lost their lives due to this largely ignored condition.

Personal Case Study #10

A nursing mother brought her three-month-old daughter, Rachel, to see me. The child had a body rash, later determined to be a salicylate toxicity reaction. The problem began in utero when the mother was told by her obstetrician to take 325 mg. of aspirin (salicylic acid) daily to prevent abnormal blood clotting (which had caused a previous miscarriage). Rachel was born with a body rash, which became worse when the nursing mother ate any foods high in salicylic acid. Rachel also had muscle tremors and cried continuously for the first six weeks of life. Rachel slowly improved with baking soda baths and magnesium in Epsom Salt baths and supplement forms, which helped to alkalize her system. We also were careful to introduce foods slowly and no high salicylate foods were given until age two.

The mother became pregnant again when Rachel was six-months-old. The aspirin regimen was again recommended by her obstetrician, even though the obstetrician was aware of the circumstances of Rachel's salicylate problem. At my urging, and the doctor's okay, 400 i.u. of vitamin E daily (instead of aspirin) was recommended due to the high risk of aspirin vs. the low risk of vitamin E. The mother had no blood clotting problems and subsequently gave birth to a healthy, full-term male who exhibited no salicylate problems. Many times physicians will opt for a drug because they aren't aware of a safer, more natural approach. To her credit, this obstetrician now recommends vitamin E as a first approach to dealing with blood clotting problems for her pregnant patients.

Dr. Holk's Rx: Pregnancy and Infant Massage Therapy

The time of pregnancy is a time of great joy. But it can also be a time of huge transition and great stress, said Annette Chamness, instructor at the Chicago School of Massage Therapy, and certified practitioner and instructor of both pregnancy and infant massage. The use of massage therapy during pregnancy is growing in popularity as more begin to recognize the benefits of such work. Studies have shown that massage therapy may decrease levels of circulating stress hormones, helping to make delivery easier. It may also play a significant role in the increased health of both mother and child. It does facilitate good posture, helping to relieving the neck aches and backaches that accompany pregnancy.

There are two excellent training programs available for massage therapists who choose to specialize in this work. Graduates of either program will be qualified to work with you throughout your pregnancy. This type of massage requires special attention to positioning on the table and may have some contraindications depending upon your health history.

One of the best treats you can give yourself is to work with a qualified massage therapist while in labor. The use of appropriate touch during this time has been shown to reduce the length of labor, reduce the use of medication, reduce the number of C-sections, reduce musculoskeletal pain, and increase the infant Apgar score. A book by Dr. Marshall Klaus, Dr. John Kennel and Phyllis Klaus, titled *Mothering the Mother. How a Doula Can Help You Have a Shorter, Easier, and Healthier Birth*, discusses the benefits of this work in detail.

Infant massage is also a wonderful form of touch therapy that has been shown to decrease colic, facilitate improved digestion, and promote better sleeping patterns. Dr. Tiffany Field's research has shown that premature infants have increased weight gain when being treated with touch therapy. Founder of the International Association of Infant Massage, Vimala Schneider McClure, has revised her classic book on infant massage titled *Infant Massage: A Handbook for Loving Parents*. This book is a helpful adjunct to the infant touch training available through one of her certified instructors. Infant massage focuses on the bonding of parent and child and the improved interaction that results from that bonding.

All children need appropriate touch. The work of Dr. Field focuses our attention on the important role massage plays in health and healing. Asthmatic children show increased peak air flow, improved pulmonary function, and less anxiety when consistently massaged by their parents. Autistic children have been shown to respond to touch therapy with increased relatedness to teachers and decreased touch sensitivity, attention to sounds, and off task classroom behavior. Adolescent bulimic girls who received massage therapy two times a week for five weeks showed improved self-image and less depression. A study done with fathers who massaged their infants daily before bed showed improved interaction between father and child. To better understand the role that appropriate touch therapy can play in your relationship with your child, see Dr. Field's book, *Touch Therapy*. There is nothing more powerfully healing than a parent's loving touch.

To find a trained and qualified practitioner of pregnancy or infant massage in your area, contact one of the organizations listed below.

For a massage practitioner who is certified in pregnancy massage:

Bodywork for the Childbearing Years:
Kate Jordan Seminars
Kate Jordan
888-287-6860
760-436-0418

Pre- and Perinatal Massage Therapy:
Body Therapy Associates
Carole Osborne-Sheets
619-748-8827

To locate a Certified Infant Massage Instructor:

International Association of Infant Massage (IAIM)
800-248-5432
805-644-8524

☙ 11 ❧

Create A Healthy Environment

FOOD SAFETY

FOODBORNE ILLNESS

While the U.S. food supply remains one of the safest in the world, the problem of a substantial number of novel pathogens is emerging while known ones are growing resistant to treatment. Since 1942, the number of known pathogens has increased **five times**. Campylobacter was the most common cause of foodborne illness in 2000, according to the Center for Disease Control and Prevention (CDC). Including other pathogens, such as salmonella, E coli, and shigella, there were 12,631 laboratory confirmed cases of pathogen poisonings in the year 2000 alone. Foodborne illness is clearly on the rise. The CDC has identified more pathogenic outbreaks in the last three years than at any other time in recent history.

One of the reasons for the rise in foodborne illness is greater centralization and dispersion of food production. The more processed foods we eat, the greater chances of food handling errors. This spreads the contamination more rapidly and makes the problem more difficult to contain. Also, eating away from home is risky. In 1978, 18 percent of our calories from food were eaten away from home. Now, 36 percent of our calories are eaten out, and this percentage is rapidly increasing. Restaurant safety laws vary according to states, but public health departments don't have the money or manpower to routinely check food establishments more than once or twice per year. What's going on the other 363 days? For protection against foodborne illness at home, *Table I: Food Safety Survival Guide* can be very helpful.

TABLE II   FOOD SAFETY SURVIVAL GUIDE

Handling Food in the Home:

The majority of food-borne illnesses are caused by improper food handling at home each year, and each year in the U.S. about 9,000 people die as a result of food poisoning.

General Handling

Utensils: Consider using an acrylic cutting board if possible, since scratches and cuts in the wood boards can hide bacteria and food particles. Wood boards can be sanitized with chlorine bleach and water. Acrylic cutting boards can also be cleaned in your dishwasher.

Work with only one perishable food at a time. Wash the board and utensils with hot, soapy water between uses.

Cooking Tips

Use a thermometer to ensure that meat and poultry are fully cooked. Put the thermometer in the thickest part of the meat, avoiding fat and bone. Bacteria is killed when meat reaches 160 degrees Fahrenheit; poultry, 180 degrees or higher.

Don't interrupt cooking by starting the job and then finishing the rest later. Partially-cooked food can be warm enough to encourage bacterial growth.

Food Storage

- Chill leftovers as soon as possible and at least within two hours of eating.
- Thaw frozen foods in the refrigerator, by placing the frozen package in a watertight plastic bag in cold water and replacing the water often.
- To protect other foods from germ-carrying meat juices, put meats in separate plastic bags at the store and then on plates before refrigerating.
- Foods that start out cold, such as opened lunch meats, should be wrapped in plastic or aluminum foil before storing.
- To cool hot foods, run cold water over sealed containers before refrigerating so the food reaches ideal storage temperature sooner.
- Store eggs inside the refrigerator compartment, not on the door compartment, because eggs need to be kept cold and often the door is not as cold as the rest of the refrigerator.
- Freezing will stop bacterial growth in certain foods, but only extreme temperatures when cooking will kill bacteria.
- Refrigerator should be set to 40 degrees or below and the freezer should be kept at 10 degrees or below. Verify temperatures with a thermometer.

Brown Bag Lunch Tips

Perishable meats or dairy products should be frozen (they'll defrost by lunch); or a frozen drink (in paper or plastic) should be added to the sealed bag.

Usage Dates to Ensure Freshness

FOOD	REFRIGERATOR	FREEZER
Poultry		
Uncooked	1-2 days	9 months
Cooked	3-4 days	4-6 months

Food	Refrigerator	Freezer
Meat		
All fresh meats		
(steaks, chops & roasts)	3-5 days	6-12 months
All ground meat	1-2 days	3-4 months
Lunch Meats		
Prepackaged, unopened	2 weeks	
Opened	1 week	
Deli meats, sliced & handled	3-4 days	1 month
Seafood		
Raw lean fish		
(cod, flounder, sole)	1-4 days	6 months
Raw fatty fish (salmon, perch)	1-2 days	3 months
Raw shrimp	4 days	3 months
Cooked seafood	3 days	2 months
Dairy		
Uncooked eggs in shell	3 weeks	
Hard-cooked eggs in shell	1 week	6 months
Milk	5 days	1 month
Mayonnaise (opened)	2 months	

*QUICK TIP:
For information about meat and poultry safety in the United States, call the FDA at 202-720-2791.
For answers about seafood, call the FDA's hot line at 1-888-SAFE FOOD.
For general information, call 202-720-2791.

Sources:
-American Public Health Association
-United States Department of Agriculture
-Food and Drug Administration

Food safety used to be the number one nutritional focus in public health. I am concerned about the fact that the most urgent nutritional challenge during the twenty-first century will be **obesity** (*Nutritional Reviews*, Volume 57; No. 12: 369). If we consequently downplay food safety, our children may or may not be thinner, but their risk for degenerative disease will certainly increase.

Preventing pesticide exposure

- Did you know that each year more than 100 million pounds of pesticides are used in U.S. homes, yards, day care centers, and schools?

- Did you know that the use of routinely used pesticides has increased at least 50 percent in the last thirty years?
- Did you know that of the 48 commonly used pesticides, 21 are known to cause cancer, 27 can adversely effect reproduction, 31 are nervous system poisons, and 17 can cause birth defects?

Pesticide toxicity through food, air, and water poses particularly serious long-term health risks for children. A landmark study of preschool children who were exposed to pesticides since birth compared to unexposed children was published in 1998 (*Environmental Health Perspectives*, June 1998, 347–53). There were no confounding variables such as genetic, dietary, or cultural differences. The pesticide exposed children demonstrated decreases in physical and mental stamina, fine eye-hand coordination, short-term memory, and ability to draw a human. What was even more alarming to the researchers was their increased unprovoked violence and aggression against parents and siblings.

The Environmental Protection Agency (EPA) was mandated in 1996 by the U.S. government to build a new margin of safety into the legal limits for 10, 000 pesticide uses, looking for the first time at neurotoxicity risks for children. So far, the EPA has only finished half of their job. How many more U.S. children will suffer physical, mental, and emotional damage before toxic pesticides are removed from our children's environment?

To protect your children from over-exposure to pesticides:

- Choose organic foods whenever possible;
- Soak fruits and vegetables in a baking soda rinse (¼ cup baking soda for every 2 quarts of filtered water);
- Don't use pesticides for your lawn and garden; encourage your neighbors to do the same;
- Don't spray your house or allow your child's school to be sprayed for vermin; there are many safer natural products;

- Drink and bathe in filtered water whenever possible;
- Write letters to the EPA and your representatives/senators in Congress to demand action against pesticide exposures.
- Use safe household products for laundry, dishwasher, and all-purpose cleaners. See the Appendix for a list of Safe Household Products.

IS YOUR HOME CHILDPROOF?

Parents are usually conscientious regarding childproofing for their infants and toddlers, but often ignore the risks to their curious children ages 4–9. Be sure to keep all chemicals and medications out-of-reach of your children and in childproof containers. Keep ipeac syrup on hand to induce vomiting quickly, if necessary. Activated charcoal (available in health food stores) has recently been shown to remove toxic foods quickly. Keep this on hand also. Always call your local poison control center for further advice if your child has swallowed a potentially dangerous substance. Make sure the poison control center number is posted where parents and caregivers can access it quickly in an emergency. Other emergency numbers should also be easily accessible.

Keeping guns away from your children should be a high priority. Among a recent survey of gun owners, 57 percent said they don't keep firearms in a locked compartment, and 30 percent admitted to having loaded guns at all times. At the risk of sounding too political, I feel that the best gun control practice in your house is NO GUNS when children are present.

WATER SAFETY

IS MY DRINKING WATER SAFE?

Local drinking water in the United States may be contaminated at many levels and in many ways. Under the Safe Drinking Water Act (governed by the EPA), Maximum Contaminant Levels (MCLs) **are** enforceable.

Eighty standards have been set. All testing is performed for single contaminants, when it is known that combinations of contaminants are usually much more volatile than single contaminants. Only public water systems are tested. Personal wells are exempt. Potential water contaminants are as follows:

- Microbes (bacteria, viruses, parasites);
- Inorganics (including lead, copper by-products, arsenic);
- Pharmaceutical and personal care products;
- Volatile organic compounds (from industrial chemicals and solvents);
- Chlorine is a double-edged sword; it disinfects but can also be toxic (Chlorine was used as a nerve poison during World War I); it is a xeno estrogen (an estrogenic cancer-causing agent).

Very few large cities have been exempt from drinking water "scares." For instance, when the filtration plant failed in Milwaukee, Wisconsin in 1993, one hundred people died and thousands became ill from cryptosporidium. Due to the heavy publicity regarding health risks of drinking water from our taps, many Americans have opted for bottled water.

Is bottled water safer than tap water?

Although the annual sales of bottled water have tripled in the last ten years, bottled water regulations are **weaker** than city tap water regulations (see Table II: Bottled vs. Tap Water Requirements).

The cost to the consumer is 250–10,000 times that of tap water. About 25 percent of bottled water is actually tap water. If the water is obtained from a deep spring and the supplier shows intermittent independent assays to prove safety, the water may be excellent. I also recommend imported waters, due to superior safety measures in European countries. Because contaminants may also leach

TABLE II: BOTTLED VS. TAP WATER REQUIREMENTS		
	Bottled Water	**Large City Tap Water**
E coli & recalcoliform banned	No	Yes
Volatile organic compounds?	1/year	4/year
Safe source or filter?	No	Yes
Disinfection required?	No	Yes
Parasite/virus testing?	No	Yes
Testing frequency?	1/week	100s/month

Sources: *Environmental Protection Agency Primary Drinking Water Regulations,* 2000
EPA Safe Drinking Water Hotline (1-800-426-4791)
NOHA News, Summer 2001

into the water from plastic bottles, I prefer glass bottles, imported, or from safe, deep springs.

The most cost efficient method of ensuring safe drinking water is to filter tap water, if high in mineral content, with a reverse osmosis carbon filter. If you community's water has a low mineral content, delivery of filtered water coolers from a decent mineral source in large glass bottled containers for home or office would be acceptable. For further information regarding safe drinking water, including what to look for in bottled or filtered water, contact: *www.cspinet.org/nah/water.*

WHAT ABOUT WATER SAFETY FOR BATHING AND SWIMMING POOLS?

If your tap water at home has a high level of chlorine, I recommend a whole-house water filter or a less expensive shower filter to remove chlorine. The skin is the largest organ in the human body. Excess chlorine exposure through the skin is as harmful as drinking chlorinated water. You will also be amazed at how much smoother and moister your hair and skin will feel by avoiding the effects of chlorine.

To prevent being exposed to excess chlorine from swimming pools, rinse off immediately upon exiting the pool, especially with filtered water. Many swimming pools today use bromine, instead of chlorine. It has far fewer side effects. Many pool owners are now installing salt water pools. They're only one third as salty as seawater with no rise in toxic substances. For more information regarding salt water pools, contact SAL-CHLOR USA at 877-392-0870 (*www.salchloreusa.com*).

Teach your children to keep their mouths closed in the swimming or wading pools. Not only can they swallow too large an amount of chlorine, but they can also contract gastrointestinal illness (*giardia intestinalis, cryptosporidium pervam, escherichia coli*, etc.). I have counseled many children who have picked up these pathogens from swallowing pool water.

SUMMER SAFETY

C. Everett Koop, M.D. and former U.S. Surgeon General, is the chairman of the not-for-profit national SAFE KIDS campaign to report data regarding seasonal injuries and to provide safety tips to prevent them. Following are some of the most important ones from SAFE KIDS and other health related organizations:

WATER ACTIVITY SAFETY

If parents begin to teach their children safe summer habits at an early age, the habits will be well established by the time they are allowed to play outdoors alone. Tips to protect your children during outdoor water activities are as follows:

- Teach your children to swim as soon as they are able. Until they become strong swimmers, never take your eyes off of them for a moment, even if a lifeguard is present. Although the American Pediatric Association disagrees with this recommendation, not panicking in water and having the ability to kick to the side of the pool could save your child's life. Children are not developmentally ready for formal swimming lessons until after their fourth birthday, states an updated policy from the American Academy of Pediatrics (AAP). According to the AAP, drowning is a leading cause of unintentional injury and death in the pediatric age group. In the United States, drowning rates are highest among toddlers ages one through two years old. In Arizona, California, Florida, and Texas, drowning is the leading cause of unintentional injury and death in this age group. While an estimated 5 to 10 million infants and preschool children participate in aquatic programs, these should not be promoted as a way to decrease the risk of drowning, the AAP says. It also says parents should not feel secure that their child is safe in water or safe from drowning after participating in an aquatic program. Whenever infants and toddlers are in or around water, an adult should be within an arm's length, providing "touch supervision," the AAP states.

- Teach your children to never swim alone. Drowning is the most common cause of summer death for children aged 14 and under. The "buddy system" could save their lives.

- Teach your children not to dive anywhere that is too shallow or where they don't know what is beneath the water.

- If you have your own swimming pool, never allow children to swim without adult supervision. Also, keep your pool gate locked to prevent young children from falling into an unsupervised pool. Consumer Products Safety offers a publication for pool safety tips. It can be accessed on the internet (*www.cpsc.gov/cpscpub/pubs/359.html*).

- Avoid beaches that are gathering spots for ducks and geese whose droppings may be harboring pathogens.

- Avoid ponds or any body of water that is stagnant.

- Avoid beaches for 24–28 hours after a heavy rainfall due to higher bacteria counts.

- Never allow your children to swim in pools or at beaches that are closed for whatever reason.
- Teach your children to rinse off with filtered water as soon as they exit a beach or pool.

Skin and eye safety in the summer sun

For optimum vitamin D absorption, allow your children to have sun exposure for 20 minutes (especially early in the morning or late afternoon) without sunscreen. At other times, apply at least SPF 15 sunscreen and lip balm to protect them against sunburn even on a cloudy day. If the sunscreen isn't waterproof, reapply as needed. Applying zinc oxide for high burn areas, such as the nose, is also helpful. Encourage your child to wear sunglasses for eye protection.

Other summer safety tips

Because nearly half of all unintentional injury-related deaths occur during the summer months, teach your child basic summer safety tips.

- **Food:** they should never eat perishable food that sits in the heat or sun for about 20 minutes or more to protect against foodborne illness.
- **Extra fluid:** extra fluids, especially water, should be encouraged when your children are playing outdoors in hot weather. Children may become dehydrated easily without even realizing it. If you allow your child to drink water from a special cup or bottle all-year around, the habit will already be established by summer.
- **Over-heating:** never leave a child alone in a car with the windows closed for even a few minutes on a warm day. The temperature can soar quickly.
- Be aware of the symptoms of **heat exhaustion:**
  pale/clammy skin
  heavy perspiration
  dizziness

weakness
headaches
cramps
nausea
fainting*

- Be aware of the more serious symptoms of
  heat stroke:
    excessively high body temperature (usually
       102 degrees or higher)
    hot, red, dry skin
    rapid pulse
    confusion and delirium
    loss of consciousness*

- **Bug bites:** flies, mosquitoes, bees, hornets, wasps, and other biting insects can quickly ruin summer fun. Some insects, especially mosquitoes, feast on people who produce excess lactic acid. To prevent bites, take Vitamin B_1 daily (doses of 25–100 mg., depending on weight, should be protective). Topical repellents, that contain no more than 10 percent DEET should also be okay, but make sure your child doesn't have a sensitivity by applying the repellant to a small area first.

    If your child is bitten, there are many natural remedies to encourage rapid healing and less itching. If the bug bite leaves a stinger, a natural way of removing the stinger and reducing swelling includes a paste of straight monosodium glutamate (MSG) with water. If your child has trouble breathing or the swelling is severe after being stung, contact your child's physician or the emergency room for further instructions.

- **Bicycle Safety:** unless your children are old enough to understand and follow all of the bicycle safety rules established by your state or local government, they should not be allowed to ride alone.

---

*See a doctor immediately or call the paramedics.

Personal Case Study #11

Robby was a very thin, allergic five-year-old child. He had been a client of mine for three years. His severe digestive distress of recent origin and one week of constant diarrhea prompted his mother to seek medical attention. The pediatrician sent a stool sample to the laboratory. It came back negative. The mother then brought Robby to see me.

I explained that it could take two to three stool samples before a pathogen is detected. After the third sample, Giardia was diagnosed. Robby had been in Florida during spring vacation where he gulped pool water. This was the suspected source.

Normally, Flagyl® (a prescription medication) is given to treat Giardia, but with highly food allergic children, it is not the best choice because it can irritate the bowel so much that it increases their incidence and severity of food sensitivities. With his pediatrician's and allergist's approval, Robby was given Uva ursi with probiotics. Both are natural pathogen destroyers. I also recommended a short-term "BRAT" diet, including binding foods such as banana, rice, applesauce, weak tea (we used a tea containing Pau d'arco because it kills pathogens) and well-cooked turkey (instead of toast to give Robby some protein). His mother made homemade chicken soup also. He ate the homemade chicken broth with rice.

I also made sure that Robby had a pediatric electrolyte drink. Contrary to popular belief, soft drinks, juices, and Gatorade® are poor electrolyte choices and may worsen diarrhea.

The diarrhea stopped after a few days, but Robby's digestion wasn't normal for a week. As he improved, we added more foods individually. He was able to stop the Uva ursi remedy after one month, but I kept him on the probiotic because it helps protect against pathogens. Three subsequent stool samples showed no Giardia and his symptoms were completely gone.

DR HOLK'S RX: REMEDIES TO "RELIEVE THE STINGS OF SUMMER"

Here are some natural tips for the bumps and bruises of life. Natural remedies and techniques can bring quick results to wounds without the unwanted side effects of prescription and over-the-counter medications. Natural remedies act to support the body's own healing process.

MINOR CUTS, SCRAPES AND WOUNDS

- Clean and disinfect the wound with soap and water to remove any dirt or debris. Lemon juice or calendula tincture (diluted five parts water to one part tincture) are excellent disinfectants as well. Calendula ointment or calendula, echinacea and goldenseal tea (cooled and swabbed on the wound), can also be used for washes of minor open wounds.

- If redness and swelling surround the wound, apply a poultice of grated raw potato and echinacea (stewed in warm water). Apply poultice directly to the wound for half an hour. Repeat as needed.

- For any trauma, wound, cuts, scrapes or falls, Arnica 200K (available only through a homeopathic or naturopathic practitioner) is an excellent homeopathic remedy, which helps reduce severity of symptoms. Give this immediately following the injury.

- Consider Bach Flower Remedy "Rescue Remedy" if your child is confused, upset or frightened.

- If your children get panicky, loses control or gets emotionally confused, give Aconite 30C.

Caution: If your child experiences numbness and tingling that does not subside or if the wound is large, deep and bleeding profusely, apply direct pressure to the wound and take your children immediately to your local emergency department.

SPRAINS AND STRAINS

- R.I.C.E.

  Rest: any motion that elicits pain should be avoided.

  Ice: Apply ice or a cool washcloth to the injured area. Cold compresses should be intermittently taken off the wound to avoid overexposure. A good formula is 2–5 minutes on, 10–20 minutes off up to 24 hours depending on the severity of the contusion.

  Compression: wrap the injury with an ace bandage making sure to apply support without causing diminished circulation to the area.

  Elevate: elevate injured limb above the level of the heart to help slow bleeding.

- Consider Arnica 200K for any trauma to the body, including sprains.

- If there is a bruise, use homeopathic Ledum 30C, especially if the bruise was caused by a blow and is cool to the touch.

- Vitamins that help with muscle and ligament repair include vitamin C, vitamin E, calcium, magnesium and manganese.

- For sprains and strains that are slow to heal and/or bone bruises, try homeopathic *Ruta graveolens* 30C.

- For muscles and joints that are stiff in the morning and better with movement and warmth, give *Rhus toxicodendron* 30C. Epsom salt baths (magnesium sulfate) are also very soothing.

- Consider acupuncture by a qualified practitioner immediately after the injury.

Caution: It is important to get sprain/strains evaluated by a qualified medical practitioner to determine the extent and cause of damage. Proper treatment may include physical therapy, an often necessary component to healing sprains/strains permanently.

Poison Oak/Ivy/Sumac

- Application of cold compresses for twenty minutes every few hours can soothe and decrease swelling.
- Apply aloe vera to the rash three to four times a day.
- Use *Rhus toxicodendron* 30C three to four times a day until symptoms lessen. This is "homeopathic" poison ivy and can be used on a daily basis until symptoms subside.
- Baths containing oatmeal (one cup to a tub of water), baking soda (a half cup to a tub) or sage tea (four ounces of herb brewed in a quart of water and strained) can soothe itching.
- Poultices of wheat bran, bentonite clay or goldenseal (diluted 5 parts water to tincture) can relieve itching. Vitamin E oil, lemon juice, cooled sage tea, and slippery elm powders or a paste of baking soda are all good applications to help soothe itching.
- Give your child plenty of fresh vegetable juices, especially carrot juice. Calcium and magnesium, vitamin C, pantothenic acid and vitamin B-complex help reduce symptoms and speed healing.

Caution: Extreme cases should be evaluated by a qualified health practitioner. In rare cases, complications can be dangerous and potentially life threatening.

Minor Insect Bites and Stings

- See "Minor Cuts, Scrapes and Wounds" for basic wound care.
- For bee stings, take Apis 30C immediately after being stung. Redose two to three more times throughout the day. This remedy will reduce the hot, burning symptoms associated with bee stings. Apis will also relieve the itching that will develop following the burning stage.
- Bee stings are very painful and often frighten children. Use Bach Flower Essence "Rescue Remedy" to help calm frazzled children.

- Apply a baking soda compress (mix baking soda and a small amount of water to form a paste) directly to the wound. To remove the stinger, use meat tenderizer made into a paste with water and applied directly to the bee sting area.
- For bites and puncture wounds take Ledum 30C. Repeated doses throughout the day are recommended. This remedy is also useful with bee stings.
- For minor insect bites a cold compress may be applied.
- Magnesium and calcium help relieve the pain of a bad bite or sting. Vitamin C and bioflavonoids help reduce inflammation and toxicity.
- Plenty of fluids, spring water and light soups can aid in flushing out toxins.
- To relieve itching, apply calamine lotion to the affected area.

Caution: Some bites and stings can cause severe symptoms and need emergency medical attention. Spider bites (black widow, brown recluse) that contain venom can cause a reaction that requires immediate emergency care.

In rare cases, an anaphylactic allergic response to bee stings can cause swelling and closing of the respiratory tract causing death. If your child is severely allergic to bee stings, seek professional medical advice to obtain emergency equipment to administer immediately after a bee sting.

SUNBURN

Caution: Sunburn is a first-degree burn of the skin. Precautions should be taken to NEVER expose your child to the point of sunburning the skin. Repeated, severe sunburns in children have been linked to higher incidences of skin cancer as an adult. Remedies to soothe sunburn:

- A mixture of half milk and half cold water makes a soothing compress.

- Beta-carotene, vitamin C, zinc and bioflavonoids for two weeks following a sunburn will help heal the skin.

- Aloe vera is very soothing and cooling to burns.

- Homeopathic *Urtica urens* will reduce the stinging, burning symptoms of sunburn. Recommended dosage is one dose of 12X or 6C every fifteen minutes for a total of four doses then one dose every hour for three more doses.

- Soaking in a cool bath will help lessen pain and cool down inflammation. Apply aloe vera gel after the bath.

- *Ferrum phosphoricum* 12X or 6C can be given every hour (up to four doses) if your child develops a slight fever.

Caution: severe sunburn can cause blistering of the skin and increase the risk of infection and dehydration. Children can get dehydrated quickly posing a life-threatening situation. Know the signs of heat exhaustion and seek immediate emergency medical care if necessary.

~❦~12~❦~

Provide Nutritional Support
for Athletes

DOES MY CHILD NEED SPECIAL FOODS FOR SPORTS?

Children and teens involved in sports, or any other stren-
uous activities on a daily basis, have to pay special attention to nutritional requirements so as not to compromise
their health or growth. This chapter will focus on the
ways in which child and teenage athletes can stay
healthy, strong, and alert.

Are there special calorie, carbohydrate, and fat needs
for athletic children and teens?

Energy needs typically depend on the child's age,
height, weight, and activity level. Usually normal weight
boys, ages 11–14 should consume about 2,500 calories/day
and girls 2,200 calories/day with about 25–30 percent of
calories from protein, 40–50 percent of calories from carbohydrate, and 25–30 percent of calories from fat.
Teenagers may require more calories, minerals, proteins,
and fats during growth spurts. Depending on the type of
training and athletic event, more calories will typically be
required.

Low carbohydrate diets are associated with fatigue and
a decrease in muscle glycogen and a decrease in
performance. If carbohydrate intake is decreased to below
20 percent of total caloric intake, glycogen stores are
compromised and, therefore, cause a lack of performance.

Fat is essential for growing children, but consuming
too much fat can lead to obesity, heart disease, and other
severe diseases. However, eating too little fat during periods of growth will not provide adequate amounts of
energy and other essential nutrients such as zinc, calcium, vitamin B_{12}, iron, magnesium, and folic acid. Diets

that reduce amounts of dietary fat and cholesterol too much tend to reduce the amount of protein and micro-nutrients that are essential for growth.

Current data has shown that consuming diets consisting of 32 percent to 55 percent fat increase endurance levels better those that only consume 15 percent fat. If fat intake is less than 20 percent of total calories, performance is compromised (*Journal of the American College of Nutrition*). For child and teen athletes, who need fat for growth, optimum brain function, and energy, adding fat during athletic training is essential. My recommendation is to include nutrient-dense fats (nuts, seeds, olive and nut oils, avocado and fish fats) for at least half of the athlete's daily fat intake. The rest of the fats can come from the foods they would typically eat.

WHAT IS A HEALTHY SPORTS DIET?

Healthy sports diets may vary, but should always balance carbohydrates with fats and/or protein for consistent energy. An example of a well balanced, nutrient-dense diet (with at least 50 percent of the fats being nutrient-dense) for a normal or underweight teen male and female athletes would look like this:

NORMAL/UNDERWEIGHT TEEN MALE

Breakfast: 3 oz. nitrate-free smoked salmon, ham, lean Canadian Bacon or ¾ cup lowfat cottage cheese
1–2 hard boiled eggs
1 fruit serving
1 waffle, pancake, or 1 small potato with small amount of butter or non-hydrogenated margarine
water

Mid A.M. Snack: ½ cup nuts/seeds with ¼ cup dried fruit
water

Lunch:	6 oz. lean beef or turkey, burger on 2 slices wholegrain dark pumpernickel or 7-grain bread with mustard, tomato, lettuce 1 cup baked veggie chips, OR 2 cups air-popped popcorn raw veggies 1 fruit serving water
Mid P.M. Snack:	toasted pita or tortilla with melted cheese OR yogurt (soy, goat's, lamb's or cow's milk's) with fruit OR hummus OR guacamole with veggies. water
Dinner:	6–8 oz. fish, lean meat, or poultry 2 cups pasta or rice (with olive/nut oil or non-hydrogenated margarine) 2 cups cooked green vegetables and/or large salad (with olive or nut oil based dressing) avocado (optional) water
Dessert:	Frozen fruit smoothie with fruit and yogurt or fortified soymilk

Note: An overweight teen male athlete may follow the above example by reducing portion sizes slightly and choosing only one snack or dessert

NORMAL/UNDERWEIGHT TEEN FEMALE

Breakfast:	2 oz. nitrate-free smoked salmon, Canadian bacon, lean ham, or ½ cup lowfat cottage cheese 1 hard-boiled egg 1 fruit, waffle, pancake, or small potato with a small amount of butter or non-hydrogenated margarine water

Mid A.M. Snack: ¼ cup nuts/seeds with 2 T. dried fruit
water

Lunch: 4 oz. lean beef or turkey burger on
1 slice dark pumpernickel bread
with mustard, tomato, lettuce
1 cup baked veggie chips, 2 cups
air-popped popcorn, or 1 fruit
¼ cup guacamole or hummus for dip
with raw veggies

Mid P.M. Snack: nut butter in celery stalks or with fruit
slices OR one mozzarella stick with
nutty rice crackers
water

Dinner: 4–6 oz. fish, lean meat, or poultry
1 cup pasta, potato, or rice (with
olive/nut oil or non-hydrogenated
margarine)
2 cups cooked green vegetables and/or
large salad (with olive/nut oil based
dressing)
avocado (optional)
water

Dessert: 8 oz. frozen fruit smoothie with fruit
and yogurt or fortified soy milk.

Note: An overweight female teen athlete may follow the above example by choosing only one snack or dessert

WHAT ARE THE BEST FLUIDS FOR MY ATHLETIC CHILD/TEEN?

Fluids play a critical role in maintaining optimal health and performance for child and teen athletes. It is crucial that an adequate amount of fluid is taken in before, during, and after each athletic activity. Fluid replacement beverages should be readily accessible for athletes to optimize oral hydration. For children and teens I recommend a **personal** water bottle for safety reasons and for optimizing the type of fluid for the individual athlete.

Sports drinks may be beneficial for replenishing fluid and carbohydrate levels if the activity is more than two hours. The quickly absorbed sugar found in the drink acts as a temporary replacement for carbohydrate loss. Avoid soft drinks, fruit punch, or caffeinated drinks because they may cause more urine production leading to dehydration. Also make sure that your sports drink is free of food dyes and artificial sweeteners.

The amount of fluid consumed during an athletic activity should be based on the rate of fluid lost through sweat and urination. In order to figure out how much fluid your child loses during an activity, it is best to weigh your child before and after exercise. For every pound lost, he or she should replenish with 16 oz. of fluid. Plain filtered mineral or spring water is the most economical source of fluid. However, your child may be willing to drink more fluid if it contains flavor. Mixing one cup of water with ¼ cup real fruit juice such as orange or pureed banana will give flavor with the added benefit of potassium and magnesium for an after game energy boost. High water fruits, such as watermelon and grapes may also be helpful. It is important to replace fluid and energy stores within one hour of high intensity sports activity. "Junk foods," such as doughnuts, cookies and canned soft drinks are poor choices. Super athletes may benefit from a sports drink that contains magnesium, potassium, and sodium in the proper ratios. Some sodium is necessary to promote thirst and to enhance fluid retention. Sports drinks should contain more potassium than sodium, and magnesium must be present in the sports drink or as an added supplement to restore or maintain electrolyte balance (refer to Table for comparisons of various common sports drinks). This is why, with the exception of Endura, HydraFuel, and UltraFuel, most of the sports drinks will not adequately restore or maintain electrolyte balance.

Comparative Content of Sports Endurance Drinks (Per 8 oz.)			
Product	Sodium	Potassium	Magnesium
*Metagenics Endura	48 mg	87.5 mg	86.5 mg
Gatorade	100 mg	30 mg	0
Powerade	22 mg	12 mg	0
Sobe Sports System	15 mg	0	0
Arizona Total Sports	100 mg	30 mg	0
*Twinlab Ultrafuel	27.5 mg	49.5 mg	12.5 mg
*Twinlab Hydrafuel	25 mg	49.5 mg	12.5 mg
Knudsen Recharge	25 mg	50 mg	0

* Recommended

HEAT RELATED ILLNESSES

Heat related illness, including heat exhaustion and heat stroke, is a serious problem for all athletes, but especially for children. It is more of a problem for prepubescent athletes, however, because they sweat less, generate more heat, and acclimate to temperature changes more slowly. They may also be less likely to recognize heat stress and dehydration before these problems become acute. Supervisors of young athletes should consider more breaks, less intensity, decreased duration of play, and more water breaks in hot weather. Parents should also help their children recognize the signs of heat illness (see Chapter 11 for details).

IMPORTANCE OF NUTRIENT-DENSE FOODS FOR CHILD & TEEN ATHLETES.

Young athletes need to eat regularly by not skipping meals and never missing breakfast, according to Jessica Donze, a pediatric nutrition therapist at the Alfred I. Dupont Hospital for Children in Wilmington, Delaware. Fruits and vegetables for adequate vitamins and minerals should be encouraged. New foods, different combinations of foods, and more minimally processed foods should be explored. An example is choosing baked potatoes instead of potato chips or a piece of fruit instead of a "fruit candy." It is important to keep young athletes interested in colorful foods. Fruits and vegetables with a lot of color are not only pleasant to the eye but also tend to have an abundance of vitamins and minerals. A powerhouse of hard-to-get nutrients are found in the following easy-to-fix snacks:

- Fortified cereal topped with banana slices or raisins/ yogurt or calcium fortified soymilk & almond or sunflower seeds
- Yogurt smoothies: 1 cup yogurt blended with 1 cup of pureed fruit (add ¼ cup of almond or peanut butter for long-term energy)
- Apple slices dipped into peanut (or almond) butter with a dash of pure maple syrup
- Toasted pita or tortilla topped with melted low fat white cheese and vegetables
- Cashew, peanut, or almond butter snack: blend 2 T. nut butter with 1 tsp. fruit spread and spread on thin cut rye toast or two rye crackers
- Banana shake: blend ¾ cup of plain cow's, rice or soy milk, 1 small banana, ¼ cup of cottage or ricotta cheese (optional), 1 tsp. honey or pure maple syrup, dash of cinnamon, and ice chips to taste (cocoa powder may be added for extra flavor)
- Well mashed tuna, egg, or salmon salad on mini rice or rye crackers
- Nut butter in celery sticks
- Frozen fruit smoothie: 8 oz. pureed fruit & 2 oz. water or juice, with 15–20 gm. whey, egg, or soy protein powder; mix altogether and freeze until firm
- Frozen banana: peel bananas; dip into cocoa or carob powder and a dash of honey or pure maple syrup; roll in ground nuts or peanuts, freeze individually in plastic wrap
- ¼ cup dried fruit with ¼–½ cup nuts/seeds. This mixture can be eaten as is or pureed with soy, whey,

or rice protein powder to make your own sports bar
(can be frozen).

- Guacamole or humus dip with vegetable or baked
corn/veggie chips
- Sports bars with a 40-20-20 ratio (40 percent mostly
complex carbohydrates, 20 percent non-hydrogenated fat, and 20 percent protein) are the best
choices. Check brands carefully. Many have added
hydrogenated fats, refined sugars, or harmful food
additives.

WHAT ABOUT EATING DISORDERS FOR CHILD AND TEEN ATHLETES?

Encouraging your children to participate in sports is
valuable for self-esteem, good health, and fun, but it is
not uncommon that the pressure to perform can be mentally and physically challenging to the child. The percent
of athletes who develop eating disorders is on the rise. If
your already underweight child or teenager loses more
body weight with athletic activity, does not eat enough
food to replenish calorie loss, or begins losing muscle
mass, parents should see this as a red flag.

The American Anorexia/Bulimia Association estimates
that more than 2 million Americans, mainly teenage girls
and young adults, suffer from an eating disorder. Preoccupation with weight has been attributed to the depic-
tion of model thin women and girls on television and
cultural values of Americans. Physically active adolescent
girls and young female athletes often eliminate animal
protein, especially meat, because they think it is fattening
and want to maintain a low body weight. By doing this
they risk protein, iron, magnesium, calcium, zinc and B_{12}
deficiencies leading to premature osteoporosis and amenorrhea (loss of menstruation).

It is essential that parents and coaches are educated
about these risks and are able to detect warning signs.
Meatless diets may be a sign of a potential problem for disordered eating. By not getting enough protein or iron in

the diet, changes in immune function, cognitive performance, concentration, body temperature, energy metabolism, and work performance can occur. Avoiding meat and
fish can also reduce zinc intake and may not meet the 15
mg. daily requirement for children ages ten and older.

Anorexia nervosa, bulimia nervosa, eating disorders
(unspecified), and anorexia athletica are the four major
types of eating disorders. Anorexia athletica is the newest
class of eating disorders which is defined as one who exercises constantly and is totally pre-occupied with diet and
body weight. The warning signs are as follows: the child
has an intense fear of gaining weight, thinks they are
becoming fat although very lean, loses weight due to
severe restriction in calorie consumption, has incorpor-
ated strange eating patterns or habits, is not menstruating,
and restricts the amount of food consumed even though
exercising extensively. Binge eating is common with purging techniques, such as vomiting, taking diuretics and/or
abusing laxatives being used to quickly remove the excess
fluid.

The combination of events, which include **eating
disorder, amenorrhea, and osteoporosis**, have been
dubbed the female triad. It is seen most often in elite
female gymnasts, runners, figure skaters, and dancers
(Warren, M.A. Stiehl, A.L, *Journal of American Womens
Association*, 1999). Because children are reaching puberty
as early as age nine and ten today and elite athletes begin
training earlier and earlier, it is even more important for
coaches to be aware of eating disorders. Life-long bone
loss and permanently stunted growth are the results of
eating disorders.

Male wrestlers, long distance runners, and body
builders are more prone to eating disorders than are males
participating in other sports. This is due to both an obsession with muscle-building and striving for a certain body
type, and possibly entering these sports due to an eating
disorder. High personal self-expectations, pressure from
their coaches, persistence, perfectionism, independence,

competition, and set goals can lead to an eating disorder that is hidden through participation in sports.

It is very important that parents and coaches take the initiative in order to prevent the onset of an eating disorder. Parents can take action by arranging a meeting with their child and his/her coach that is both supportive and confidential.

Any athlete suspected of having an eating disorder should be referred to a multidisciplinary health care team trained in eating disorders with an expertise in sports-related eating disorders. It is also an excellent idea for coaches to bring in speakers to talk about sound nutritional practices for athletes and to debunk ideal body weights for certain sports.

WHAT DIETARY SUPPLEMENTS SHOULD MY ATHLETIC CHILD OR TEEN TAKE?

My supplement recommendations vary greatly depending upon the child's age, growth rate, and type of athletic activity. As mentioned previously, I almost always recommend magnesium. Magnesium is the most important nutrient for muscle and heart metabolism, nerve transmission and relaxation, synthesis of genetic material within each cell and the conversion of fats, carbohydrates, and protein to energy. Ideal food sources for magnesium include avocado, kiwi, nuts/seeds, soy products, bananas, oranges, salmon, halibut, mackeral, unsulphured and blackstrap molasses, and cocoa powder.

Almost 75 percent of people living in the U.S. are magnesium deficient. Athletes lose magnesium with workouts, so I recommend high magnesium foods and supplementation of magnesium for almost all of the child and teen athletes I counsel. I also recommend regular Epsom salt (magnesium sulfate) baths. Although potassium is usually the focus of sports nutritional requirements, it is usually easy to get enough from food. Without adequate magnesium, however, potassium won't be readily absorbed.

I almost always recommend a good multi-vitamin and mineral formula that includes the U.S. Government recommendations for iron, zinc, and trace minerals. Unless a child is not ingesting 800–1000 mg. of calcium from food regularly, I usually do not recommend extra calcium. Contrary to the obsession most Americans have with calcium, especially from milk or calcium carbonate supplements, getting too much calcium causes mineral imbalance, reduced magnesium stores, and poor absorption of calcium. I have seen dozens of teen athletes consuming 2000 mg. or more of calcium daily who were shocked to discover that their bone spurs, muscle cramps, and stress fractures were caused by too much calcium and too little magnesium. Balance is very important. Through acquiring most of their nutrients from food, children/teens will benefit by adding nutritional supplements for total body conditioning (see Chapter 14 for specific supplement recommendations).

WHAT DIETARY SUPPLEMENTS SHOULD MY ATHLETIC CHILD OR TEEN NOT TAKE?

Child and teen athletes should not take Ephedra or Ma huang. These dietary supplements cause the heart to race, and have been known to cause serious heart arrythmias and even death. Creatine, a "muscle building" amino acid, should never be taken by children or adolescents because no tests have even shown that it is safe taken in supplement form (*Journal of the American Academy of Pediatrics*, August 2000). The American College of Sports Medicine discourages its use for anyone younger than age eighteen.

Personal Case Study #12

Fifteen-year-old Michael and his parents came to see me because Michael "short circuited" and felt such low energy on the basketball court that his coach told this super sophomore athlete that he would be kicked off the varsity team if he did not fix the problem. Michael's pediatrician ruled out any medical condition and referred him to me.

Michael ate a typical "junk food" diet with lots of soft drinks. The sports drink he consumed regularly at basketball practice and games seemed to make him feel worse. He told me he was willing to try anything because "basketball is my life."

My dietary recommendations were similar to the ones highlighted in this chapter for an underweight athlete. I also supplemented his diet with magnesium, B-vitamins, Co-Q$_{10}$, zinc, and a high potassium electrolyte drink before and after workouts, practices, and games.

Our session was on Tuesday. By that Friday evening's game, he played almost the entire game. His coach couldn't believe the difference in his energy level and concentration. Two years later, I had the privilege of watching Michael on television as he led his high school to a third place victory in the Illinois State basketball championship.

DR. HOLK'S RX

Athletes should never take energy enhancement supplements, other than vitamins and minerals, unless under the direction of a licensed health professional who has expertise in sports nutrition. Some supplements, such as Ephedra, Ma huang, and Creatine, should never be used by children or teen athletes for energy, endurance, or building muscle mass. A safe energy and endurance substitute for teens who weigh more than one hundred pounds is Co-Q$_{10}$. According to the *Physician's Desk Reference*, "*CoEnzyme Q10 (Co-Q$_{10}$) is an essential cofactor in the mitochondrial electron transport chain, the biochemical pathway in cellular respiration from which ATP and metabolic energy is derived. Since nearly all cellular functions are dependent on energy, Co-Q$_{10}$ is essential for the health of all* *human tissues and organs."* (*Physician's Desk Reference*, 1992, page 2377) Taking 30 mg. before practice or a sporting event can optimize the athlete's cellular energy to minimize fatigue.

Chromium can help build muscle and burn fat. It also helps to regulate insulin. Most athletes over one hundred pounds can safely take 100–200 mcg. daily after their first meal of the day. Also, taking magnesium in a glycinate (glycine) form will help build muscle mass even more than magnesium in an oxide form because **glycine** is required for synthesis of naturally occurring creatine, which helps slow degeneration of muscle tissue.

❧ 13 ❧

Determine Your Child's Food and Chemical Sensitivities: The Oligoantigenic (Elimination) Diet

In the 1980s, Joseph Egger performed a brilliant study for what he called the "hyperkinetic syndrome" in children (Egger, 1987). He reviewed in detail the therapies that were presently in use (i.e., psychostimulant drugs, behavioral approaches, and the Feingold diet). He determined that **medicated** children show no long-term benefits either in social or academic areas; and although drug treatment may increase the time spent focusing on a task, it does not necessarily improve task performance. (Egger 1987, p. 676). With regards to **behavioral therapy**, he agreed that it could help in the short-term, but there is no evidence of a long-term effect. One of the flaws of this approach is that many of the parents who would be required to use the behavioral techniques with their children have too many problems of their own for assured compliance to the program (Egger, 1987, p.676) The Feingold Diet, an additive-free, salicylate-free plan, showed benefit with a small subgroup of children; and in the future it could show significant promise for treating hyperkinetic children (Egger, 1987, pp. 676–8).

Joseph Egger's review of the literature showed that since early in the 20th century, the role of **food allergy** had often been suspected with regards to the hyperkinetic syndrome and that a number of studies confirmed this notion. He, therefore, decided to perform a study of his own with a very restricted four-week oligoantigenic (elimination) diet (see Table 1) since he determined that

TABLE I OLIGOANTIGENIC DIET CHOICES

Ideal Diet	Alternate Diet
Turkey	Lamb
Cruciferous vegetables (cabbage, brussel sprouts, cauliflower, broccoli)	Carrots, Parsnips
Potato (and potato flower)	Rice (and rice flour)
Banana	Pears
Soy Oil	Sunflower Oil
Water (filtered)	Water (filtered)
Salt	Salt
Calcium and multivitamin (additive-free)	Calcium and multivitamin (additive-free)

Reference: Eggers, 1987

any food could be a potential allergen. If improvements occurred during the elimination phase, he would use a double-blind provocation technique that would reintroduce one food at a time. If there were no improvements during that elimination phase, it was assumed that the patient either did not comply or was not food intolerant.

He noticed some very interesting phenomena during the strict diet phase. First, most children went through a few days of worsened symptoms due to withdrawal reactions. Second, the reactive foods were most often not the foods that the children disliked, but usually the foods eaten most frequently and often craved. Third, not only did hyperkinetic behavior diminish during the elimination phase, but other complaints of headache, fatigue, restlessness, sluggishness, irritability, and abdominal pains disappeared while interest in school, work, increased concentration, and play improved considerably. Although children complained about the diet, they liked the way they felt after the withdrawal phase ended.

Joseph Egger's results were dramatic. The diet proved more beneficial for hyperkinetic children than did medication and behavioral techniques combined. The oligoantigenic diet has now become a valuable tool for other related health problems including migraines, digestive disorders, and chronic upper respiratory infections. Many versions of the oligoantigenic diet since Egger's study have been used, including shorter duration, and modified versions that allow for greater compliance.

I have experimented with many versions of an Elimination Diet in the last eighteen years. I use it mostly as a tool to prove to families that dietary changes can make a noticeable difference in their entire family's physical, mental, social, and emotional well-being. The diet usually can pinpoint the following major imbalances:

- Yeast imbalance/Tyramine foods
- Salicylate toxicity
- Gluten (the "glue" in most grains) intolerance
- Casein (milk protein) and/or lactose (milk sugar) intolerance
- True allergy to specific foods
- Erratic blood sugar (due to excess carbohydrate and too little protein intake)
- Some children have exhibited only one of these imbalances; others have exhibited all of them. I have only seen two cases where no improvement occurred when the elimination diet was followed correctly.

When we identify an allergy as the main problem, I refer to a board certified allergist for further testing. If we suspect a gluten intolerance problem, I refer to a gastroenterologist for a digestive diagnosis. If any of the other results occur and further testing is necessary, I often refer to a preventive physician who uses a wide variety of techniques to clinically diagnose offending foods.

It is important that the entire family follows the diet together. It is also helpful if families embark on this program with the assistance of a knowledgeable licensed health professional who can encourage them through both the elimination and provocation stages to be watchful for any problems that might arise. For assistance in finding a health professional who may be familiar with elimination diets in your area, contact The Certified Board of Nutrition Specialists/American College of Nutrition at (727) 446-6806 or *office@cert-nutrition.org*, or the American Dietetic Association for names of licensed nutrition experts in your area.

The following **Modified Oligoantigenic Diet** shows the greatest family compliance because it is "kid friendly" and because it identifies specific brands (available at natural food stores) that are quick to prepare. I also recommend an added dietary magnesium supplement (or Epsom Salt bath), added Calcium (additive-free), and adequate protein and fat. This plan is very healthy because it contains adequate protein, contains no hydrogenated fats, and contains good amounts of essential fatty acids, and trace vitamins/minerals. I don't usually recommend a multi-vitamin/mineral until we discover which foods are reactive. The best part of the food plan is that the foods are minimally processed, nutrient-dense and additive/sugar-free.

MODIFIED OLIGOANTINGENIC (ELIMINATION) FOOD PLAN

It is important to follow this plan exactly for 14–21 days. If a brand name is mentioned, only that brand may be used. Carbohydrates must be limited and never should be eaten alone (must be accompanied by a fat and/or protein). Proteins and fats are unlimited, as long as a minimum of each is consumed to regulate blood sugar.

Please note: If any of the following items have shown past reactions, delete them from the list.

LIMITED FOOD PORTIONS

Carbohydrates: Daily Maximum ___4 ___5 ___6 (The usual recommendation is 4 carbos for an overweight child, 5 for a normal weight child, and 6 for an underweight child)

Grain/grain substitutes	Vegetables/Vegetable Snacks	Fruits
8 oz Rice Cream (original lite or enriched plain only)	1 medium sweet potato or yam	
5 small Hain rice cakes (plain) or Edward & Sons rice crackers (plain)	spaghetti, acorn or butternut squash	1 whole organic sweet apple
¾ cup plain brown or converted rice (no rice mixtures)	1 medium white potato (preferably Yukon Gold)	1 whole Asian pear
Puffed Rice cereal	artichoke (fresh or canned in salt water	1 whole banana
Cream of Rice cereal	carrots	1 whole pear
¾ cup China Bowl Cellophane noodles (pea/potato starch)	Jicama	½ cup canned pears, in juice, drained
1 slice Ener-G yeast free rice bread	brussel sprouts	½ guava
¾ cup quinoa	cauliflower	½ mango
¾ cup Pastariso, DeBole's or Lundberg's rice pasta	green peas	1 slice watermelon
	green or yellow wax beans	½ small papaya
	1 cup Cascadian Farms or or homemade baked french fries	6 oz. pureed fruit from any fruits listed above (add water to make a smoothie)
	1 cup Kettle or Michael Season' potato chips, plain	
	1 cup Barbara's sweet potato chips	

Proteins: Daily Minimum ___3 ___4 ___5 (**minimum depends on age**; children 5 and under would have 3 portions minimum; children 5 to 8 would have 4 minimum; children 9 and up would have 5 portions minimum)

   2 oz. organic, free-range or Kosher turkey
   2 oz. organic, free-range or Kosher chicken
   2 oz. Cornish hen
   2 oz. lean duck
   One Pork Shop of Vermont uncured beef frankfurter

2 oz. organic, free-range or kosher lamb
2 oz organic, free-range or kosher beef
2 oz. organic deli turkey breast
2 oz. lean organic pork (chops, tenderloin)
One Yorkshire Farms turkey frank
3 oz. Spence & Co. or other brand of naturally
    smoked salmon
3 oz. poached/broiled/baked salmon, halibut, mackerel
3 oz. sardines, canned (packed in water or olive oil)

Fats Daily Minimum ___2 portions **minimum**
¼ whole avocado
1 T. extra virgin olive oil
8 black olives (cured in water/salt only)
1 T. Spectrum margarine
1 T. sunflower oil
1 T. rice bran oil
¼ cup pepitas, pumpkin or sunflower seeds
    (raw/dry roasted)

UNLIMITED FOOD CHOICES

(The following foods are unlimited unless otherwise stated)

Condiments/Spices (fresh/frozen/dried)	Vegetables	Other
garlic	celery	mineral water (plain or sparkling, filtered)
onion	organic lettuce	Green Leaf Stevia Plus with F.O.S. (non-caloric sugar substitute)
parsley	endive	any brand of Stevia (no other ingredients)
sea salt/kosher salt	kale	
chives	radicchio	
shallots	escarole	
leeks	bok choy	
saffron	hearts of palm	

After the 14–21 day strict elimination phase, we begin the provocation phase by adding categories of foods (always the least suspected, least craved foods first to the most craved last). If a food is never eaten by your child and won't be "hidden" in processed foods, that test may be deleted. Following are the categories I use to test (waiting 4–7 days between categories). If there is a reaction to any test in any category, wait 7 days, then start the next category.

Categories: Because many of these foods are found in more than one category, it is best to choose foods found only in the category being tested.

- **Salicylate Foods**

  (1st) **Moderate** (test at least 2 from this category on the same day): almonds, apricot, beets, blueberries, broccoli, cucumber (with skin), dates, eggplant, figs, ginger, honey, lime, mushrooms, mustard powder, pimiento, red/yellow cooked peppers, rice wine vinegar, saffron, spinach, tangerine/tangelo, vanilla, weak green/black tea, wintergreen, zucchini

  (2nd) **Strong** (if no reaction to moderate, test at least 2 from this category on the same day): allspice, almonds, anise, basil, bayleaf, cinnamon, citric acid, fruit spread, grape, grapefruit, mint (peppermint, spearmint) orange, oregano, paprika, peanut, pepper (black, chili, red, cayenne), pickles, plum, prune, raisin, raspberry, strawberry, blackberry, red wine/ balsamic vinegar, rosemary, strong coffee, tarragon, tart apples (i.e., Granny Smith), thyme, tomato (fresh, juice, sauce), bell peppers (raw), wine, champagne

  (3rd) **Other Salicylates** (more potent than food salicylates; testing not recommended unless under the direction of a physician):

  Yellow dyes #5 & #6, red dye #40, BHA/BHT, nitrates/nitrites, caramel color, any cola

  Any medication containing aspirin or an aspirin cross-reactor (check with a physician or pharmacist for further direction). **Never give a child aspirin.**

- **Yeast/Tyramine Foods**

  (1st) **Moderate** (test at least 2 from this category on the same day): barbecue sauce, carrot/beet juice, canteloupe, honeydew melon, catsup, cornstarch, dried fruit, grapes, herbal teas (containing grass/pollen derivatives), cashew nuts, pistachio nuts, ice cream, kefir, non-organic milk, yogurt, non-organic meats or poultry, miso, soymilk with added sugar, tempeh, tofu, flat breads (flour tortilla, pita)

(2nd) **Strong** (if no reaction to moderate, test at least 2 from this category on the same day): aged cheese (especially blue and aged cheddar), beer, champagne, wine, chocolate (bittersweet/milk), fruit juice (especially apple, grape, orange), high sugar foods (candy, cake, cookies), mushrooms, naturally fermented sauerkraut, peanuts/peanut butter, pickles, sorbet with added sugar, soy sauce, vinegar (especially wine, balsamic), yeasty bread (especially very fresh)

- **Legumes** (excluding soy): start with carob powder; next alfalfa sprouts; organic white beans; next red or garbanzo beans; finally lentils, split peas and dry roasted peanuts or peanut butter
- **Soy Foods:** start with soy lecithin/oil; next tofu; next soymilk (less than 10 gm. sugar); tempeh; next soy nuts/edamame; finally soy protein powder
- **Citrus:** start with lemon; next lime; next grapefruit; next citron/tangerine/tangelo; finally orange
- **Tree Nuts** (test each one on separate day): test ¼ cup of any desired nuts (i.e. pine nuts, walnuts, pecans, hazelnuts, almonds, Brazil nuts)
- **Eggs** (use only organic brands): start with one egg the first day; if tolerated 1 yolk with 3 whites can be tested on the next day
- **Dairy Products:** start with butter or full fat cream; next mozzarella or Farmer's cheese; next cottage or ricotta cheese; next yogurt; next aged cheeses; and finally milk (use organic or imported brands only)
- **Fish/Shellfish** (test every fish desired on a separate day): test any desired coldwater fish first; next lake fish; finally, shellfish
- **Grain/Gluten** (excluding corn): start with Arrowhead Mills Puffed Millet; next Arrowhead Mills or Erewhon

instant (plain) oatmeal; next Ryvita or Wasa (no yeast) rye crackers; next barley; next any durum or semolina (i.e., couscous, pasta); finally plain whole wheat cereal (i.e., shredded wheat) or plain whole wheat crackers (i.e., Wasa wheat)

- **Corn:** start with plain cornflakes or grits; next baked corn chips; next plain popcorn; next corn syrup or high fructose corn syrup; finally cornstarch as a thickener (1 teaspoon per person maximum)

The symptoms that are most common when a food is added back are as follows:

Elimination Diet® Symptoms when Adding Back Foods*
- Weight gain (if your child is overweight)
- Fluid retention/edema (fingers, toes, ankles, face and/or joints become swollen)
- Gas/bloating (stomach becoming distended with or without flatulence)
- Stomachache, nausea, vomiting, diarrhea, abdominal cramping
- Fatigue for no explainable reason
- Irritability, aggression, anger, or nervousness
- Headache
- Attention problems or hyperkinetic (agitated) behavior
- Red ears and/or cheeks
- Skin break-outs (rash, bumps, hives, pimples)
- Itching
- Depression/lethargy for no explainable reason
- Asthma attack or breathing problems (contact your physician immediately)
- Flu-like symptoms
- Congestion/excess mucus production (runny nose, sinus, throat, or lung congestion)

***WARNING:** if your child has asthma or has ever had any breathing problems or seizures, contact your child's physician before testing any foods.

It is very important to keep a detailed list of reactions so that your licensed health professional can assist you in deciding what further tests, if any, may be necessary. If a category shows no reactions, it is considered acceptable and may be added back into your child's diet.

I have personally seen dramatic improvements (physical, mental, social, and emotional) through elimination diet testing. Some of the most dramatic changes have been stopping chronic diarrhea, headaches, and total body rash or itching in days. As I tell my clients, 2–3 weeks out of an entire lifetime to assess food connections related to health conditions is something anyone can try!

Personal Case Study #13

Two-year-old David's holistic physician referred him to me to see if there was a nutritional connection to his painful, itchy body rash. Herbal treatments and avoiding environmental triggers had helped 60–70 percent. I told David's parents that often my elimination diet parents have as much success as do their children. David's mother said the whole family would follow the diet to offer support to David, although she knew she had no food sensitivities. She thought her husband might benefit because he was always tired, congested, and had a hand tremor that puzzled medical experts.

The elimination diet revealed milk and yeast sensitivities for David, a salicylate sensitivity for the mother, and milk, yeast, and wheat sensitivities for the father. David's father ended up being more delighted than anyone because his chronic congestion, fatigue, and even his hand tremor disappeared.

ꄿ14ꄾ

Give Complete Nutritional Support to Your Kids

VITAMIN SUPPLEMENTATION FOR KIDS IS NOT A LUXURY, IT IS A NECESSITY

Now that half of America's kids consume less than the recommended daily allowances for four key minerals – zinc, iron, magnesium, and calcium – rickets (a vitamin D deficiency) has started to make a comeback, nutritionists are becoming alarmed. Infant formula companies are now even fortifying foods that toddlers will eat; namely, cookies and crackers.

I have always been uncomfortable recommending a "one size fits all" approach to nutritional supplementation whether in supplements or foods. The following recommendations include the nutrients necessary to prevent the common deficiencies of most American children.

INFANCY

- **Iron:** Iron deficiency is an ongoing dilemma. During the past 30 years, there has been a dramatic increase in iron deficient anemia during the first year of life. Supplemental iron (the ferrous form) for breast-fed babies after six months of age, either as a liquid or in fortified infant cereals, is essential. For formula-fed infants, iron fortified formulas should be given until age one.

- **Vitamin D:** This should be taken after six months for breast-fed infants in liquid, fortified foods, or sunlight exposure (20 minutes early morning or late afternoon several times per week) without sunscreen.

- **Cod Liver Oil:** This is one of my favorite sources of vitamins A & D during winter months because it nourishes mucus membranes, boosts the immune system, and is a natural source of DHA (see DHA section). If your infant (six months and older) will not take cod liver oil orally, applying it topically will absorb almost as well (½ tsp. orally/1 tsp. topically). For vegan breast-feeding mothers, I recommend cod liver oil all year around.

- **Liquid Multiple Vitamin:** An infant multi-vitamin supplement containing A, B, C, D, E, and K should be taken after formula or breast-feeding stops.

- **Probiotics:** Probiotics should either be taken by the breast-feeding mother (lactobacillus acidophilus and bifidus) or given in small doses to infants who are formula-fed to stimulate their immune system, minimize allergies, and aid digestion and absorption. A recent double-blinded study in the *Journal of Pediatrics* found that infants who were given probiotics, particularly lactobaccili, had an 80 percent lowered risk of developing diarrhea compared to other infants (*Journal of Pediatrics*, 2001; 138: 361-5).

- **EFAs:** Essential Fatty Acids (EFAs) in the form of safflower oil, are now found in some baby formulas. There are also supplement preparations containing concentrated EFAs from safflower that may be added to baby formulas. *Warning:* I do not recommend fish oil EFAs for children until one year due to allergen potential.

- **DHA and AA:** These should be added to infant formulas if not already present. Breast-milk is already naturally rich in these substances. Docosahexaeonic acid (DHA) and Arachidonic acid (AA), both long chain polyunsaturated fatty acids which are found naturally in breast milk, are not found in most infant formulas. These fatty acids enhance mental and visual development in infants and play a pivotal role in brain function throughout life. Cod Liver Oil is a natural source of DHA. If a child is under one year of age, I recommend organic high oleic safflower oil in capsule or liquid form.

TODDLERS AND YOUNG CHILDREN (AGES 2–5)

Toddlers and young children (through age 5) are typically not meeting Dietary Reference Intakes (DRI) in the United States of iron, zinc, calcium, magnesium, vitamin A, vitamin B_6, and vitamin D. These nutrient shortages in early childhood have adverse consequences that may be only partially reversible. Iron deficiency, in particular, affects about 15 million children and is linked to long-term impairment of brain function, attention span, intelligence quotient, and school performance. Low calcium, vitamin D, and magnesium levels may cause childhood rickets and prevent peak bone mass in adulthood. Dietary Reference Intakes are **minimum**, not **optimum** requirements.

Our Paleolithic ancestors consumed 5.8 times as much iron, 2.7 times as much zinc, 1.6 times as much of the other micronutrients as do modern humans owing to the predominance of micronutrient rich, unprocessed foods such as meat, root vegetables, nuts, and fruits in their diet. Because American children will not realistically adopt a Paleolithic diet, supplementation of these nutrients is essential to prevent long-term health consequences and to reach optimum nutrient levels. When supplementing with any vitamins or minerals, make sure they are free of artificial colors, flavors, harmful preservatives, and known allergens.

- **Zinc:** Zinc is deficient among most of the nation's toddlers. It is a critical mineral for growth, absorption of proteins and carbohydrates, brain development, and a healthy immune system. It is so important for disease prevention that the World Health Organization found that supplemental zinc can reduce pneumonia by as much as 41 percent and diarrhea by as much as 25 percent for young children (Black, Sazawal, Shankar, *American Journal of Pediatrics*, December 2000). I recommend that all toddlers supplement with 5–10 mg. of zinc (dependent on age and size) in a liquid form or as part of a chewable multiple vitamin/mineral.

- **Iron:** The 1994 Third National Health and Nutrition Survey Report and 1998 U.S. Department of Agriculture found that daily iron intake among one to two year olds is lower than that of any other age group (only between 55 and 60 percent of recommended intake). At such a crucial time for growth, this problem has become a serious public health issue. Routine daily iron-supplementation in a liquid or multi vitamin/mineral of 5–10 mg. (in ferrous form) for all toddlers is a wiser choice than the "screen and treat" approach for iron anemia now advocated by the American Academy of Pediatrics, according to Alvin Eden, M.D., Clinical Professor of Pediatrics, Cornell Medical Center in New York *(Nutrition & the M.D.*, Vol. 27, No. 1, Jan. 2001). I agree, wholeheartedly with Dr. Eden, especially because iron deficiency can be erratic instead of constant, and even a slight iron deficiency (not clinical anemia) has adverse effects.

- **Vitamin A & D:** Supplemental Cod Liver Oil during winter months and vitamin A & D fortified rice, soy, or cow's milk year around should provide enough of these vitamins for most healthy toddlers who get adequate sunlight exposure. One teaspoon of cod liver oil daily is usually sufficient.

- **Calcium:** If your toddler takes in 16 oz. of calcium-rich rice, soy, or cow's milk, and eats one high calcium food daily (cheese, salmon, sardines, fortified tofu), this is sufficient calcium for most children. I have often seen parents so worried about calcium intake that they overdose their toddlers with chewable calcium tablets, causing imbalances of other minerals, kidney stones, artery and joint calcification, etc. If your 4–5 year old child routinely ingests less than 400 mg. of calcium daily from high calcium or fortified foods, a calcium chewable of 250-500 mg. or less would be acceptable.

- **Magnesium:** Seventy-five percent of all people living in the U.S. are magnesium deficient. Since magnesium is a catalyst for over three hundred bodily functions, including behavior, concentration, and serotonin balance, I almost always recommend supplementing young children's diets with 100 mg. of highly absorbable magnesium (such as Magnesium Glycinate). Magnesium, in a glycinate form, doesn't usually cause a loose bowel problem (if your child is routinely constipated, magnesium oxide or aspartate may be preferable). If your child cannot tolerate oral magnesium, Epsom Salt baths (2–4 cups of salts per bath), which contain magnesium sulfate, will provide some magnesium absorption if given four or more times weekly.

- **B Vitamins:** B-complex vitamins found in most toddler multiple vitamin preparations for young children are usually adequate doses for healthy children. If your child has special needs (see other chapters), added dosages of B-vitamins, especially B_6, B_{12}, and folic acid may be necessary.

- **Probiotics:** These are important for young children to aid digestion, strengthen the immune system, and to minimize food borne illness.

SCHOOL AGED CHILDREN (AGES 6–11)

In the past, school-aged children have typically been healthier than young children, especially if school-based feeding programs exist. The school cafeteria should be a learning laboratory for food choices. Unfortunately, with the introduction of fast foods and vending machines in school lunchrooms, the quality of school cafeteria food choices has deteriorated.

Nutritional deficiencies have devastating consequences for school-aged children, including absenteeism, poor school performance, and behavioral problems. Deficiencies of iron, vitamin A, calcium, magnesium, and zinc appear to be the most pronounced. Because schools are a "captive audience" for nutrient additions during lunch, it would make sense for the U.S. government to mandate the availability of multi-vitamin and mineral supplements (based on DRIs) for all children. The cost-benefit ratio of this type of "feeding" program would be incredible.

In the absence of supplemental nutrients added to school lunches, I recommend that 250 mg. of calcium, 100 mg. of magnesium, 15 mg. of zinc, 10–18 mg. of iron, 2500 i.u. of vitamin A (in the form of beta carotene), 200 i.u. of vitamin D, 30 i.u. of vitamin E, 100 mg. of vitamin C, 200 mcg. of folic acid, 10 mg. of B_6, and 25 mcg. of B_{12} routinely be given in supplement form to most healthy 6–11 year old children. Some of these levels are higher than the DRIs, but I feel they are necessary for optimum physical, mental, and emotional function.

TEENAGERS (Ages 12–18)

The teen group needs more nutrients for rapid growth than does any other age group except 1–3 year olds. At a time of sexual and linear growth, **zinc** is the most critical nutrient for males, while **iron** may be the most important nutrient for menstruating female teens. In fact, one recent study performed at the University of Rochester found that even mild iron deficiency can lower math test scores (Hlaterman, *J. Journal Ped.*, June 2001). This may explain why teen girls often score worse than teen boys in math, even though their scores are usually similar in elementary and middle school.

I recommend a teen formula (there are many well-balanced ones found through licensed health professionals or in health food stores) that includes the following for most healthy teens:

- **Calcium:** 200–400 mg. (more if the teen's food calcium intake is less than 500 mg.)
- **Magnesium:** 200-300 mg.
- **Vitamin D:** 400 i.u.
- **Zinc:** 15 mg. (up to 30 mg. for teens who exhibit short stature, chronic colds, and acne)
- **Iron:** 15 mg. (up to 36 mg. for females who are anemic or who have heavy menstrual periods)
- **Vitamin A:** 2500 i.u. from fish oil (or **none** if the teen uses a topical Vitamin A acne formula)
- **Vitamin A:** 5000 i.u. from beta carotene
- **Vitamin C:** 150-500 mg.
- **Vitamin E:** 100-200 i.u.
- **Vitamin B$_1$:** 25-50 mg.
- **Vitamin B$_2$:** 25-50 mg.
- **Vitamin B$_3$:** 25-50 mg.
- **Vitamin B$_6$:** 25-50 mg.
- **Folic Acid:** 400 mcg.
- **Vitamin B$_{12}$:** 50-200 mcg.

In addition, I would add the following probiotics:

- **Lactobacillus Acidophilus:** 1 capsule or ¼ tsp. powder (if active culture yogurt is not eaten regularly)

Although I always recommend eating **real food** as the first line-of-defense for building health, I realize that nutrient losses and sub-optimal dietary habits are probably going to be the norm for many children and teens. Therefore, government mandated vitamin and mineral supplements added to foods they enjoy, or supplements (free of artificial colors, flavors, sugar, hydrogenated oils and allergens) given by their conscientious parents, should provide the best "health insurance" we could buy for our American youth.

LET'S GO BACK TO GETTING MOST OF OUR NUTRIENTS FROM REAL FOOD

WHAT DOES IT MEAN TO EAT REAL FOOD?

The USDA Food Pyramid is a disaster. For 1.6 million years our Paleolithic ancestors lived on wild game, seafood, fruits, vegetables, and nuts – all gathered in the wild. There were **no grains** and **no dairy** products. A mere 10,000 years ago, when an ever-growing human population and food scarcity forced humans to cultivate grains to prevent starvation, our farming ancestors showed marked signs of malnutrition, manifested in loss of height and increased incidence of disease. Expert geneticists claim that agriculture is too recent for our nutritional needs to have changed genetically more than 0.05 percent since Paleolithic times (Simopolous, A., *Genetic Variation and Nutrition*, 1999).

Unfortunately, we have had even more drastic changes in our food supply since the advent of World War II, especially in the United States. Essential fatty acids have been replaced with heavily saturated and hydrogenated fats. Over-processing of our foods has depleted nutrient levels to such a low level that even the USDA is now recommending fortification of vitamins and minerals to foods that toddlers will eat.

The vast majority of children's food products are disasters. *If manufacturers were trying to undermine children's health, they could hardly be more effective*, said Dr. Tim Lobstein, co-author of a year 2000 Food Commission Report. *There is a huge opportunity to promote healthy products to children using all the marketing tricks of the trade . . . but, instead, we are seeing unhealthy ones being promoted* (Lobstein, T. Food Commission Report, 2000). Food manufacturers are interested in shelf life, not **your** life. Profit is the name of the game. If a food has a shorter shelf life, it usually is less profitable. If anyone had told me that a popular brand of cupcakes on my office shelf would still look like cupcakes 18 years later, I would not have believed it. If you don't believe it's possible, do your own experiment with your favorite processed foods. If a real food is real, it will get rotten quickly! If a food lasts weeks or months, it is probably so laden with chemicals and preservatives that even bacteria won't want to feed on it.

WHAT CONSTITUTES JUNK FOOD?

For decades, dietitians have insisted that there are no real junk foods, just unhealthy diets. Well, times have changed. Prestigious nutrition journals and the National Health and Nutrition Examination Survey (*NHANES*) have determined that one-third of America's diet is made up of "junk food," described as energy-dense, nutrient-poor foods that don't belong in the major food groups of fruit, vegetables, meat/meat substitutes, grains, or dairy products. Some of these junk food culprits include:

- visible saturated/hydrogenated fats (butter, margarine, lard, gravies);
- sweeteners (sugar, syrup, candy, sweetened beverages);
- desserts (cookies, cakes, cupcakes, pastries, ice cream, pudding);
- salty snacks (hydrogenated potato, corn, and other chips or snack crackers);
- miscellaneous (artificially colored/flavored diet drinks, and candies).

Ashima Kant, PhD., Associate Professor of Nutrition at Queens College in New York, says *such patterns of eating take both a nutritional and health toll. The higher the intake of junk foods, the lower is the likelihood of meeting current recommendations for a healthy diet or having adequate intake of important vitamins and minerals* (Kant, A. *JAMA* 2000; 283: 2115). The lifelong consequences are increased incidence of disease and earlier death from any cause.

Soft drinks are probably the most prominent junk food source. More than 15 billion gallons, one-fourth of all drinks consumed daily, were sold in the U.S. in the year 2000. Kids are heavy consumers; 56 percent of all eight-year olds in the U.S. drink soft drinks daily. One-third of U.S. teenage boys drink at least three cans of soft drinks daily. The consequences are a sharp rise in obesity (for each serving of a sugar-sweetened soft drink daily, the risk of obesity increases 1.6 times), more tooth decay, bone weakening (increasing the risk of osteoporosis at earlier ages), and caffeine dependence.

Toddlers who consume junk food are at very high risk for cavities and more serious problems, including stunted growth and poor school performance. Toddlers who consume candy and sweetened juice more than once a week at age three are nearly twice as likely to have cavities by age six, compared to their peers who eat sweets no more than once a week (Karjalainen S. *Dentistry & Oral Epidemiology* 2001; 29: 136-142). Researchers have known for years that the toddler stage is a "window-of-opportunity" for cell growth, especially in the brain. If adequate nutrients are not received or depleted by eating junk food, the brain may never function to its full potential. However, is it prudent, as Mead Johnson believes with their Enfagrow® products, to put vitamins and minerals into cookies and snack crackers for kids? I would much rather teach healthy eating habits by introducing real foods.

What if junk food manufacturers had to pay a "junk food tax?" What if the money could go to fund healthy food and dietary supplement programs for impoverished children? Or better, what if the public had to pay a higher tax for junk foods that contained warnings such as:

> WARNING:
> This food contains hydrogenated oils (or) high levels of refined sweeteners which the Surgeon General has deemed a high risk for degenerative disease.

This way, people who eat healthy foods will not be as burdened by skyrocketing taxes and health insurance rates to compensate for people who pay no attention to building their health.

One policy that **can** and **must** be changed, is peddling junk food to kids in schools. Vendors of soft drinks, candy, chips, and other nutrient-poor foods are enticing schools to use sales of these foods during school hours to raise money for school activities. Schools should not have a financial interest in promoting junk food. Parents need to demand of schools that our children's mental, physical, and emotional health be put before profit.

WHAT CONSTITUTES OVEREATING?

If your children are eating according to the USDA Food Pyramid, they are probably overeating. But, if they are regularly eating junk food outside of the Food Pyramid, they are almost definitely overeating. Portions are another problem. Most restaurant and fast food portions are double or triple the amount recommended for one meal. Most Americans have adopted a "bigger is better" mindset (i.e., Whopper; Grande Latte, Big Mac), instead of looking at quality of ingredients.

In my practice, showing parents and children portion sizes is beneficial. Many of them are shocked to see visuals showing how small a portion really is, especially for rice or pasta. A useful guide to easily visualize food portions is to compare portions to known products. For instance:

- 1 serving of meat/poultry = deck of cards
- ½ cup rice, pasta, fruit, or vegetable serving = the fist of a small adult hand
- 1 pancake, waffle, tortilla, pita = the diameter of a CD
- 1 baked potato = the size of a computer mouse

Schools can easily teach portions sizes from pre-school upwards. One of the favorite activities of young children is playing store. With appropriate portions of a wide variety of foods being constantly used in play, conditioning may become automatic. In later years, when nutrition units are taught in science classes, portions should always be shown, studied, and tested. As I travel from classroom to classroom, I am always surprised that teaching food portions are seldom part of the nutrition curriculum.

MY CHILD IS A 'PICKY' EATER. WHAT CAN I DO?

A picky eater is made, not born. If children see their parents eating only healthful foods, that will be the norm in the household. If dad is drinking a soft drink and eating high fat chips, candy, and cookies, in front of the television, that is what your child will see as the norm. Just as with alcohol, if you don't want to encourage drinking among your teens, you don't want them to observe you drinking a "six-pack" nightly to relieve stress.

Many studies show that children who eat healthfully as infants and toddlers, adopt these principles for life. For instance, children who don't eat sugar until age two like it less and voluntarily eat less later in life. In addition, if toddlers are exposed to a wide variety of only nutrient-dense foods at home and can make unrestricted choices from these foods, they will naturally balance their calories and nutrients to meet their needs. Since self-control is a lifelong problem for food intake, this is an important concept.

Following are tips for preventing picky eating and adopting healthy eating for life:

- Be a good role model of healthful eating of a **wide variety of foods.**
- Offer a variety of foods. Even if your child first rejects a food, continue introducing it. Research has shown that exposing children to a new food ten times may be the magic number! The importance of eating variety in your diet reaches far beyond physical health. Research studies have also shown that eating a wide variety of foods at age two was a strong predictor of better scores on cognitive and achievement tests at age 11.

- Always offer protein first. Kids have no trouble getting enough carbohydrates. If they eat carbohydrates first, the protein foods will look less appealing. If they have protein first, they generally will not overeat carbohydrates.

- Do not reward or bribe children to eat or to try new foods. The more parents push or bribe, the less children may eat. Especially avoid promising dessert or junk food as a way to get children to eat healthy foods.

- Never offer juice before food. Your child's blood sugar may become so elevated that your child won't want to eat much. Because excess juice, even if it is all-natural, can contribute to obesity and prevent adequate linear growth, the new American Academy of Pediatrics guidelines for juice intake are as follows:

Age	Amount Daily
Under 1 year	No Juice
Ages 1–6	6 oz. maximum with water (diluted throughout the day)
Ages 7–18	8–12 oz. maximum

Source: *American Academy of Pediatrics, 2000.*

- Don't tell your child to avoid junk foods; they will want them even more. The best way to teach healthful eating is by keeping your kitchen stocked full of easily accessible, healthy foods. Not restricting any foods in the house (because they are all healthy) is also the best way to teach kids eating self-control early. It also is much easier for you, as parents, to not have to become a "food cop." Some parents make a special snack shelf in a cupboard and refrigerator so that children can help themselves easily. Cutting foods up into bite-size portions makes it even more convenient. When my children were young, I cut fruits, vegetables, and lowfat cheese into bite size portions and put them into sealed containers in the refrigerator for easy access.

- Teachers and parents should never use foods as rewards or punish children who choose not to eat a particular foods or a particular meal. My eating disorder clients still have nightmares about being made to sit for hours at a dinner table to "finish their peas." I even have clients who wake up in the middle of the night to eat cake or cookies because those foods were used to soothe pain and hurt of childhood events or as a reward for a job well done. Food is for nourishment of our bodies and should not be forced or withheld.

- Make sure your children eat an adequate amount of protein daily (eggs, dairy products, fish, poultry, and meat provide complete proteins). Growing children who are vegan (and don't supplement their diet) or who hate all animal protein usually lack key micronutrients (B_{12}, zinc, and iron in particular) and macronutrients (protein and essential fats). Health problems may develop from lack of bioavailable protein, including urinary tract and ear infections, chronic upper respiratory infections, obesity or failure to thrive, learning problems, and chronic fatigue. If your family is strictly vegan, it is important to have your child evaluated by a licensed health professional to ensure nutritional adequacy.

How can I handle eating situations for my child who has food sensitivities?

One of the most difficult challenges of my nutritional practice is to find alternative foods when children have multiple food sensitivities. Many of the children I counsel have reactions to cow's milk products, yeast-producing foods, gluten, corn, and wheat (i.e., the American diet). Fortunately, catalogs and natural food stores today have a plethora of tasty substitute foods. It is imperative that parents keep these on hand and avoid restriction of "safe foods" at home.

When your child eats elsewhere, parents need to provide substitute foods and explain to the adult in charge why your child cannot eat other foods. Once children are old enough to understand, they will usually be quite diligent about avoiding reactive foods because they don't want to feel sick. The problem I see more often is grandparents and friend's parents or caregivers not reading labels or reassuring food sensitive children that a "little bit" won't hurt. I have seen children rushed to hospitals because they trusted a misinformed adult. Parents can avert this problem by having their child or adult promise to call if there is a food that is offered that might be a problem.

There is a wonderful Be-a-Pal program, developed by the Virginia-based Food Allergy and Anaphylaxis Network (FAAN) for children with food allergies. The program helps severely allergic kids to stay away from allergic foods that could cause them to have a life threatening reaction. PALS are friends who agree to help their allergic friend avoid their dangerous foods. Knowing how to seek help if their friend has a reaction, avoiding their friend's allergenic foods themselves, and keeping "safe foods" in their own homes for play dates all help the severely allergic child to feel less isolated. For more information regarding Be-a-Pal, contact FAAN at (800) 929-4040 or visit their website at *www.foodallergy.org*.

THERE IS SO MUCH INFORMATION ABOUT HEALTHY EATING. IT IS OVERWHELMING. ISN'T THERE AN EASIER WAY TO LOOK AT WHAT FOODS ARE GOOD AND WHAT FOODS AREN'T?

An easy-to-follow detailed guide for healthy eating is found in my first book, *Nutrition in a Nutshell* (Vital Health Publishing, 1999). For the quickest look at how to eat healthy, *Table II* identifies *Food and Chemical Effects of Acid/Alkaline Production*. The American diet is 80–90 percent acid-forming. Excess acid, also produced by stress, medications, and environmental pollutants, is the

TABLE II FOOD AND CHEMICAL EFFECTS ON ACID/ALKALINE PRODUCTION

FOOD	Most Alkaline	More Alkaline	Low Alkaline	Lowest Alkaline
Additive, spice Condiments	Baking soda Sea salt			
Beverages	Mineral water (sparkling, plain)		Kambucha	Ginseng
Sweeteners			Rice syrup	Molasses
Vinegar				
Milk Products Cow				Ghee (clarified butter)
Soy				
Goat/Sheep				
Eggs			Quail eggs	Duck eggs
Meat				
Fish/Shellfish				
Fowl				
Grains & Grain Substitute				Rice milk Tapioca Quinoa Wild rice
Nuts, Oil & Seeds			Avocado oil Primrose oil Cod liver oil	Poppy seeds Pumpkin seeds Coconut oil, cocnut Olive oil, olives (black) Flax oil Sunflower seeds, oil
Veggies and Legumes	Seaweed Onion/Miso Daikon/Taro root Sea vegetables Burdock/Lotus root Sweet Potato/Yam	Kohlrabi Parsnip/Taro Garlic Carrots Kale/Parsley Endive/Arugula Most greens	Potato (white) Mushroom/Fungi Sprouts Cabbage Rutabaga Artichoke Eggplant Pumpkin Collard greens	Brussel sprouts Beet Chive/Cilantro Celery Okra Cucumber Squashes (orange) Lettuce (all types) Jicama
Fruits	Watermelon	Crenshaw melon Canteloupe Honeydew melon Pineapple Mango	Lemon Pear Avocado Apple (sweet) Nectarine Cherry Passion Fruit Papaya	Kiwi Apricot Banana Blueberry Peach Dewberry Loganberry Persimmon Starfruit

Sources: Jaffe, R. *Health Studies Collegium*, 2000
Buist, R. *Food/Chemical Sensitivity*. New York
Pennington, J. *Bowes & Church's Food Values of Proteins*. NY Lippincott, 1998.

Lowest Acid	Low Acid	More Acid	Most Acid
Ginger	Most spices	Cinnamon, Mustard	Food Dye, Catsup
Tamari	Coca	Benzoate/Sulfites	Black, white cayenne
Kona Coffee	Wine/Champagne	Soy sauce, Worcest.	Beer, Liquers
Green tea, Sake	Black tea	Grain/hard liquor	Yeast/Hops, Malt
Stevia	Sucralose	Coffee/Grain coffe	Sugar, white and
Maple syrup		Saccharin, Honey	brown
Rice vinegar	Baslamic	Milk chocolate	White/Acetic vinegar
	Apple cider	White	
Cream/butter	Cottage cheese	Casein (milk protein)	Processed cheese
Yogurt	Ricotta cheese	Aged cheese	Dye-containing
	New cheese	Cow's milk	Ice cream
	(Farmer's)		
Soy milk	Soy Cheese,	Soybeans	Hydrogenated
	Tofu, Tempeh	Soy nuts	margarine
Cheese (goat/sheep)	Milk (goat/sheep)		
Chicken eggs			
Turkey eggs			
Gelatin		Pork/Veal	Beef, organ meat
		Game meat	
Fish	Shellfish, Mollusks	Mussels, Squid	Lobster
Goose, Turkey	Wild duck	Pheasant	
	Quail, Chicken,		
	Cornish hen		
Oats,	Buckwheat/Kasha	Maize, corn	Wheat
Millet	White converted rice	Barley	(whole, bran, germ)
Brown rice	Spelt, Teff, Kamut	Triciale	
	Amaranth	Farina, Semoilina	Rye
	Seitan		
Grape seed oil	Almond oil, almond	Pistachio seed	Cottonseed oil
Macadamia nuts	Sesame oil, seeds	Chestnut oil, chestnut	Fried foods
Canola oil	Safflower oil	Lard	Hydrogenated fats
Soy oil	Hazelnuts, Walnuts	Pine nuts	Hydrogenated
	Brazil nuts, Pecans	Palm kernel oil	margarines
	Non-hydrogenated		
	margarine		
Radish	Pinot beans	Asparagus	
Fresh green peas	Navy beans	Peanut	
Cauliflower	Aduki beans	Snow/green pea	
Broccoli	White bean	Lentil bean	
String/Wax beans	Lima bean	Fava/Kidney bean	
Zucchini	Chard	Chick pea/Garbanzo	
Spinach	Rhubarb	Carob	
	Bell peppers		
Water chestnuts			
Guava	Plum	Cranberry	Hot peppers
	Pickled fruit	Prune	Pomegrante
	Dried fruit	Tomato	Citrus (except lemon)
	Figs	Grape	Tart apple
	Raspberry	Raisin	Tomato sauce
	Cherimoya	Strawberry	
	Dates	Blackberry	

beginning of degenerative disease and health problems. Some children typically never eat any of the alkalizing foods listed. Keeping your family's diet to about 60 percent acid/40 percent alkaline (and completely avoiding the most acid foods, if you already have excess acid), will be the most dramatic step you could take for building your family's health. Although rare in the U.S., too much alkalinity can also cause problems. Balance is the key. It is easy to celebrate the delicious colors, smells, and flavors of real foods. If every week your family would eliminate one acid food and add one alkaline food to achieve balance, the results would be dramatic.

Another great, fun-filled book I highly recommend for the entire family is the online children's book, *Fantastifood Fables: Attack of the Junk Food Junkies*. This fable about a brother and sister that have to save the Land of Fantastifood from the dastardly Junk Food Junkies is a fantastic way to learn that healthy eating is fun! The website to view the book is *http://www.fantastifood.com*.

Optimal health can be achieved through eating a real foods diet. Robert Crayhon, nutrition expert, says that *Optimal health is not the result of deprivation. It celebrates the benefits of many foods and nutrients, allowing us more of life and health. It is the marriage of science and pleasure.* **Balance** *the information to your own best advantage* (Crayhon, *Nutrition Made Simple: A Comprehensive Guide to the Latest Findings in Optimal Nutrition*, 1996).

Personal Case Study #14

Eric's mother originally came to one of my group sessions on how to implement an elimination diet. When she heard my comments, she realized that her son's asthma might be related to food sensitivities and was eager to try the diet. She decided to bring Eric in for a private session with me because she felt that at age twelve, he would respond better to my suggestions than to hers.

Eric was at least twenty pounds overweight, very large for his age, and very distracted in my office. He couldn't sit still. He said he felt stupid because he was in several learning disabled classes, was the last child into the gym when the junior high kids ran in from recess because he couldn't breathe, and was labeled by teachers as a trouble-maker. He was using his inhalers more and more with less success. His pediatrician was now recommending a fourth course of cortisone, which Eric didn't want to take because he said it made him fatter. He was constantly being teased about his weight by other children. Eric became very motivated to try the two-week elimination diet.

The first week was tough for Eric because he had to give up his favorite foods of tomato sauce, catsup, bread and diet soft drinks. He was also teased about his unusual lunches, which he told other kids was a "Sports Diet."

The second week Eric started feeling energetic and more focused in the classroom. He had not needed his inhaler more than once since the diet began. He started dropping a lot of weight (fluid build-up) and was no longer feeling the need to "act out" in class.

When he came back to see me on the fifteenth day of the diet, I didn't recognize him. He had lost twelve pounds of fluid, seemed much calmer, and was more focused. He excitedly told me that he was the first person in the gym now, and his fellow students thought his "Sports Diet" was amazing. He received the first stars of his life for five perfect days at school. The principal now called him "little man" instead of "big guy" because he was so polite. But Eric felt best about the fact that he could now easily play the drum sequence he had been struggling to learn.

Eric's supposed asthma has now been re-diagnosed by an allergist as severe allergies to corn, tomato, chocolate, and milk. No wonder he couldn't run after lunch at school without an inhaler. His breathing problem was really an anaphylactic reaction to catsup, chocolate milk, and corn tortilla chips he consumed at lunch.

Eric continues to do well three years later. He now plays drum in the high school band, is no longer in learning disabled classes, and is a starter on the freshman basketball team. Many of his friends have asked him for advice so they, too, can follow his "Sports Diet."

ᕽ‍C 15 ᑉ

Enhance Your Child's Emotional I.Q.

WHAT IS EMOTIONAL I.Q.?

Emotional I.Q.s, unlike Intelligence I.Q., shows how well your child is able to cope in a variety of situations, including at home, with peers, in school, and in extra-curricular activities. Parents are so often preoccupied with building their children's intellectual skills and over-loading them with out-of-school activities, such as play-ing a musical instrument, taking art classes, and toddler organized sports, that time is not allotted for the child to merely "be a child." In 1981, the average school-aged child had 40 percent of the day for free time (not engaged in sleeping, eating, studying, or organized activities). By 1997, this figure dropped to 25 percent. Play doesn't just make kids happy, it makes them smarter.

Asked in a recent study what skills children needed in order to be prepared for school, teachers cited social skills, such as sharing and interacting with others, and following instructions as the most important. *Intelligence is based on emotional adequacy*, says child-development expert, T. Berry Brazelton. *The concept of emotional intelligence is at the base of all this.* (Brazelton, T. Berry, M.D. *Touchpoints: The Essential Reference.* New York: Addison-Wesley Publishing Company, 1992.)

SO WHAT SHOULD PARENTS SUBSTITUTE FOR BRAIN TOYS?

If interpersonal skills are the true predictors of how well a child will do in school, parents are the best tutors. Allowing children to have more play-time, under the watchful eye of parents (or of teachers and care-givers), will allow children to learn better coping skills through necessary interaction with other children. Recess during school, for instance, is a great teaching ground for learning how to cope. We used to laugh when children described recess as their "favorite subject." It is very possible that these children became the adults with the highest Emotional I.Q.

I recall my oldest son's friend in their early years of high school. The young man was a straight "A" student, gifted in math and science, and a decent soccer player. My son sometimes felt inferior to him. But the day a speech had to be given in English class, the tables turned. My son, confident and unafraid of an audience, and comfortable with his peers, gave an animated presentation, which earned him an A+ from his teacher and peers. His brilliant friend started shaking in front of his classmates, forgot his speech, and retreated in defeat. My son was flabbergasted, but realized that sometimes the high Intelligence Quotient isn't enough to make it in this world.

PARENTS NEED TO BE INVOLVED IN THEIR CHILD'S EDUCATION

Too many harried moms and dads are playing hooky when it comes to raising their kids. Schools are luring them back. But more needs to be done. When I began teaching in Cabrini Green, one of Chicago's worst ghettos in 1969, I had 35 third graders, most of whom functioned at a pre-school level. When I held parent-teacher conferences, the only parents who came were the parents of my five hopeful students – the ones who had the brains and self-esteem to "make it." I could tell that their parents believed in their child's ability to succeed and were willing to go the extra mile to make it happen.

The simple, obvious answer to "what we can do to help our kids?" is to be there through thick and thin, tell them you are there for them, help them when they fall, and give them unconditional love. It doesn't mean fighting their battles and doing their projects to make life easier for them. It means giving them emotional support to allow them to fail and helping them succeed, even if the successes are small baby steps.

There are many ways in which parents and schools can ensure parental involvement including:

- **Staying involved from pre-school through high school.** Studies show that parental involvement drops off dramatically between sixth and ninth grades. When this happens, teens become less manageable and less communicative. It is often a relief for an unsure teen, afraid of too much responsibility in a potentially dangerous situation, to be able to say, *Sorry, my parents will kill me if I do* . . .

- **Learning how to sat "no."** We are rearing a generation of kids who are enjoying outrageous excesses, becoming overly materialistic, and not being expected to be accountable for misbehavior. A priority in home and at school should be performing tasks to be "rewarded" with an allowance or special school privilege. A child who is required to participate in chores, babysit, and not be handed everything "on a silver platter" will grow up to be more self-confident and hard-working. It is frightening for a child to have no limits. A parent who is strict (but reasonable), out of love for their child, will create a responsible, loving and caring child.

- **Schools giving parents real power** such as providing parent-run school improvement teams and holding meetings so that parents can voice their concerns in an organized format.

- **Teachers being accessible.** It is important for teachers to contact parents if there is a school problem, but it is equally important for parents to contact teachers if they are concerned about their child's problems or performance. Supporting the teacher's rules and goals are essential.

- **Parents sitting in the classroom with their child for a day if they have had constant behavioral or learning problems.** There is no better way for a child to "shape-up" or for the parent to understand the reasons for their failure than if the child's parent is actively participating. Many schools also encourage parent helpers. I always opted to help in subjects in which I knew my children were having the most trouble. It improved their ability to comprehend those subjects better because I was better able to help them.

- **Schools holding parents accountable** for their child's dress code, help with homework, checking to see that homework is finished, etc. If parents have to sign "contracts" to this effect, it keeps parents involved and the child knows it.

WHAT ARE THE MOST IMPORTANT SKILLS NEEDED FOR PARENTS TO RAISE THEIR CHILD'S EMOTIONAL I.Q.?

For children, infancy through age 12, the following eight skills will make the most difference, but can be adapted to any age if you start early:

1. Building positive self-esteem. This helps your child develop an "I can do it" attitude. Tips: Encourage or reinforce positive behavior immediately when it happens; be realistic about praise (your child can spot a "fib" a mile away); expect a lot, but not more than your child can provide; avoid comparing your child to other children, especially siblings; and avoid labels such as shy, stubborn, hyper, and clumsy (it is amazing how kids have radar to hear everything you say, even when they pretend they are not listening).

2. Cultivating strengths. Point out your child's strengths only when deserved; kids know the truth. Parents can be role models by making more positive (rather than negative) statements about themselves. For instance, I always tell my children, *Show me, don't tell me. I am a visual learner* instead of *I won't remember what you tell me, I have an auditory memory problem.*

3. Communicating. Listening, encouraging, communicating, and making suggestions without judging will encourage your child's emotional success throughout life. This is one area where having a parent at home when kids get home from school (the moment that the child is bursting to discuss their day) or having the entire family adopt a dinner ritual of telling other family members about their day, will make a big difference. If your child is reluctant to communicate freely, encourage the child with questions such as *How did the math test go?* or *You have a big smile on your face. Did something great happen today?* If you discuss your child's great days often, the child will be more apt to bring up the "not-so-good" days as well.

4. Problem solving. Self-reliance is a lifelong gift. If your child has confidence that even serious problems are surmountable, emotional health will build. Teaching them a five-step approach (called STAND) for making decisions (as soon as they are old enough) is:

S = Stop, calm down, and identify your feelings;
T = Tell them what the problem is (a parent, friend, sibling);
A = Ask, "What are my alternatives?";
N = Narrow the choices; and
D = Decide on the best choice and do it.

This does not mean that family members solve the problem and take action themselves. I vividly remember a bully chasing me home from school in third grade with constant taunts and jeers. The faster I ran, the faster he ran. Some days he would even pull my pony tail. I asked my older brother to "beat up the bully" for me. He refused, but helped me find ways to solve the problem myself. I finally decided upon the "kick him where it hurts option." When I acted upon this decision the following day, the bully never bothered me again and my peers were in awe that a little girl like me could scare away a big bully.

5. Getting Along. Children who are the most popular in school are those who have enough self-confidence to smile, share, and help out other children. Having good manners, such as politeness, also helps. Allowing children to interact with dolls or action figures during play can encourage getting along. If young children show one doll or figure acting mean to other dolls or action figures, encourage the child to have them make-up or say they are sorry. Parents who admit they make mistakes and say they're sorry also help.

6. Goal setting. Children who target what they want to achieve and who take reasonable steps to achieve these goals will usually be successful. Realistic goal setting is very important. If a child says I want to be the best diver on the team, help the child begin with one dive that can be mastered and build slowly. Expecting an unrealistic goal can make a child feel like a failure. Parents should also make sure that the goal is one the child envisions, and not a parental goal for the child. I remember one of my children's friends who loved swimming and wanted to be on the swimming team in high school. His father, an ex-college football player, wanted him to focus upon football. The son solved the problem by becoming an adequate player on the football team and a star swimmer. He eventually went on to become a star swimmer in college.

7. Not Giving Up. I believe that perseverance is the most important skill for building your child's emotional I.Q. Everyone makes mistakes. Everyone has setbacks, even with ideas and projects that should be successful. University of Michigan research shows that **teaching a child to value effort** is a better predictor for success than judging innate abilities. I always encouraged my children to "follow the road less traveled" if they believed in an idea or project strongly. How many famous discoveries in our world today would not be here if the naysayers had won, those who said people can't fly . . . a man on the moon, ridiculous . . . nothing will ever replace a horse and carriage...

8. Caring. If you want your child to think about the needs and feelings of others, it is important to teach your child ethical responsibility. Parents are the ideal role models for compassion and helping out others through kind acts and deeds. This can begin with your child helping siblings, younger friends, or young cousins.

Caring supervision begins at home

It is very important for parents to be home with their pre-teens (children aged 7–12) or have adult supervision at all times when they are away from home. Most parents would be shocked to discover how many unhealthy behaviors are going on among kids in this age group who come home from school alone. Pornography, alcohol, and negative Internet sites are being used. Smoking, drinking, sex, and drug use begin earlier, sometimes calamitously, when children who are too young to be responsible for themselves are put in this position. The results of these behaviors may have serious long-term consequences. This is a time when kids are testing themselves and need strict parameters. After school clubs or sports activities for kids whose parents work during these hours can help. Don't assume that your eleven-year old can take care of your six-year old every day after school. These children don't have the skills to meet the challenges necessary to provide a nurturing, safe environment.

I have seen every pitfall of parenting . . . from wealthy parents who have been too busy with their social life to be there so they shower their kids with expensive toys . . .to workaholic parents who let the nanny raise their kids . . . to poverty stricken parents who don't have the physical or emotional energy to discipline their active children.

I may be criticized for my strong feelings, based on years of observations, but I believe that at least one parent should be on hand to raise their child for the majority of their child's waking hours each day until the child reaches high school age. Childhood flies by and those hours spent together, through good and bad times, tighten the parent-child bond, not by **teaching** but by **showing** unconditional love.

(Adapted from: Michelle Borba, *Parents Do Make A Difference: How to Raise Kids with Solid Character, Strong Minds, and Caring Hearts*, Jossey-Bass, 2000.)

CONCLUSION

Food For Thought

You, as parents, can become proactive instead of reactive when it comes to your child's physical, mental, emotional, and social well-being. According to Dr. Robert Reynolds, Associate Professor of Human Nutrition and Dietetics,

> *Nutrient deficiencies may be one of the root causes of today's oppressive crush of poverty in this otherwise affluent society. Most social programs aimed at the affected children will not, or cannot, reverse this situation. It is already too late by the time they are children. A more liberal, yet responsible, acceptance of supplementation or fortification by the government, aimed at the mother either before onset of pregnancy or in the early stages of pregnancy and continuing through lactation . . . will have a chance of being effective in reducing the impaired development of these children*

> (*Nutrition Today*, Vol. 35, No. 6, 2000: 227.)

I agree that intervening with vitamin and mineral supplements to build mental capacity and immunity before childhood will improve the U.S public health more dramatically than any effort ever proposed, except sanitation. In 1998, Senators Orrin Hatch and Tom Harkin urged ex-President Clinton to reverse the U.S. Department of Agriculture's 14-year policy prohibiting the use of Food Stamps for vitamin and mineral purchases. Poverty-stricken mothers, infants, and children are the most nutritionally deficient segment of the population. Instead of waiting for problems to set in, the U.S. Public Health Department can save money and lives by interceding **before** problems arise.

When today's students enter school with established preferences for fast foods, sweetened beverages, and heavily salted fatty foods; when students visit the school's vending machines and snack bars instead of eating a balanced meal in the school cafeteria; when obesity among children is reaching an epidemic level; and when one-third of the American diet is junk food, it is time for the U.S. government to step in. Fortunately, several public health bills have been introduced in the U.S. Congress as this book goes to press to change the status quo. They are:

- Antibiotic Resistance Prevention Act of 2001 (recommends more than 80 steps to address the growing antibiotic resistance problem);
- Better Nutrition for School Children Act of 2001 (would mandate that unhealthy food and beverages not be sold or given to students anywhere on school property during meals);
- Medikids Health Insurance Act of 2001 (would provide national health insurance to all children born after 2002; would include screening and prevention);
- Safe Food Act of 2001 (would consolidate all food safety activities into one, more powerful agency); and
- Gun Show Loophole Closing and Gun Law Enforcement Act of 2001 (would address the sale of firearms at gun shows by requiring criminal background checks at events that provide a venue for gun sales).

(**Source:** *The Nation's Health*, July 2001.)

For further information on the status of any of these bills, and what you can do to ensure they pass, visit the <Thomas.loc.gov.> website or call your state representative or senator's offices.

My goal for all the children I serve, and, hopefully your goal for your children, will include the following:

THE PRINCIPLES OF OPTIMUM HEALTH FOR OUR CHILDREN

1. A positive self image.
2. A diet free of toxic foods.
3. A diet that provides optimum levels of all beneficial nutrients.
4. Clean Air, Water, and Living Environment.
5. Adequate (but not excess) sunshine.
6. Adequate exercise and rest.
7. Safety at home, at school, and with peers.

I no longer **educate** poverty-stricken children. I no longer **counsel** learning and emotionally disabled teenagers. I do, however, continue to pursue my goal of **providing optimum nutritional support** for children and their families to promote optimum physical, mental, and emotional well-being. Hopefully, this book has given empowerment to all who have the courage to reach beyond the status quo and to be the best they can be. In the words of a child,* *Everyone has inside of him a piece of good news. The good news is that you don't know how great you can be! How much you can love! How much you can accomplish! And what your potential is!*

* Anne Frank, written while hiding from the Nazis

APPENDIX

Safe Household Products

ALL PURPOSE CLEANERS

To make your own all-purpose disinfectant & cleaner: Mixture of 2 teaspoons Borax, 4 tablespoons White Distilled Vinegar, ¼ cup of Earth Rite Dishwashing liquid and 3–4 cups hot water in a refillable spray bottle. Use pump spray only. Never use aerosols.

AFM Enterprises Safety Clean
AFM Enterprises Super clean
Arm & Hammer Baking Soda (*to deodorize*)
Aubrey Clean Up! All Purpose Household Cleaner
Auro Organics Plant Soap
Auro Organics Cleaning Emulsion
Bioclean
Biofa Household Cleaner
Bon Ami Cleaning Cake
Borax (to disinfect)
Dr. Bronner's Pure Castille Soaps
Dr. Bronner's Sal Suds (32 oz, $9.89 each)
Dr. Harvey's All Purpose Clean
Earth Rite All Purpose Cleaner (22 oz, $3.99 each)
Earth Rite Countertop Cleaner
Greenspan Healthy Kleaner
Naturally Yours Degreaser
Naturally Yours Gentle Soap
Seventh Generation All Purpose Cleaner
    (32 oz, $4.39 each)
Simmons Pure Soaps
Tropical Soap Co. Sirene Coconut Oil Bar Soaps
Vinegar (white distilled)
    especially good for cleaning windows and tile floors

BATHROOM CLEANERS & DISINFECTANTS

AFM Mildew Control
Biofa Natural Toilet Cleaner

Descale-It Bathroom Tile and Fixture
Dial Corporation 20 Mule Team Borax
Earth Friendly Toilet Cleaner (16 oz, $2.89 each)
Earth Rite Tub and Tile cleaner
Eliminate Shower Clean Tub and Tile
Naturally Yours Basin, Tub, and Tile Cleaner
Naturally Yours Mold and Mildew Cleaner
Neo-Life Green Personal Care Cleaner
Nutribiotic Drops or Spray
Spic and Span Pine

BLEACH SUBSTITUTES

Hydrogen Peroxide (*any brand*)
Naturally Yours Natural Bleach and Softener

CARPET CLEANERS & DEODERIZERS

AFM Carpet Cleaner
AFM Carpet Guard
Airwick Carpet Fresh
Bissell Wall-to-Wall Rug Shampoo
Granny's Karpet Klean Carpet Shampoo
Naturally Yours Carpet and Upholstery Extraction
    Detergent
O'Cedar Carpet Science Spot and Stain Remover
Resolve Carpet Cleaner (*pump*)
Woolite Deep Cleaning Rug Cleaner
Woolite Tough Stain Rug Cleaner

DISHWASHING LIQUIDS (HAND)

Aloe Care
Arm & Hammer Baking Soda
Arm & Hammer Super Washing Soda
Biofa Natural Dishwashing Liquid
Borax
Cal Ben Soap Company Seafoam Dish Glow
Chef's Soap
Dermassage Dishwashing Liquid
Dove Light Duty Dishwashing Liquid
Earth Rite Dishwashing Liquid (22 oz, $3.69 each)
Naturally Yours Dishwashing Detergent

Dishwashing Detergents (Automatic)

Cal Ben Seafoam Destain for Automatic Dishwashers
Kleer II Liquid
Kleer III Powder
Shaklee Basic D (*New*)
Shaklee Basic D (*Old*)

Floor Cleaners, Waxes & Polishes

Auro Organics Floor Wax-Balm cleaner
Auro Organics Plan Alcohol Thinner
Auro Organics Boiled Linseed Oil
Bon Ami Cleaning Powder
Earth Rite All Surface Floor Cleaner
Ecover Floor Soap (32 oz, $4.59 each)
Karen's Nontoxic Products (*Lemon Oil*)
Karen's Nontoxic Products (*Pine Oil*)
Livo's Avi-Soap Concentrate
Livos Kiros-Alcohol Thinner
Parker's Wood Cleaner and Floor Polish
Vinegar (White Distilled) – *not for wood floors*
Wood Finishing Supply Company (*Beeswax*)
Wood Finishing Supply Company (*Carnuba Wax*)

Furniture Polishes

Axiom Block Oil
Biofa Natural Furniture and Floor Cleaning Emulsion
Earth Rite Furniture Polish (16 oz, $5.09 each)
Naturally Yours Furniture Cleaner and Protector
Old English Wood Soap
Parker's Perfect Polish (*Butcher Block*)
Parker's Perfect Polish Classic (*Potpurri Oil*)
Parker's Perfect Polish (*Cabinet Clean*)
Parker's Perfect Polish (*Lemon Oil*)
Parker's Perfect Polish (*Wood Finish Cream*)
Wood Plus Furniture Polish and Cleaner

Glass & Window Cleaners

Cinch Glass and Multi-surface Cleaner
Earth Rite Glass Cleaner (22 oz, $4.29 each)
Dr. Harvey's Glass Clean
Natural Chemistry Glass Cleaner

Naturally Yours Glass and Window Cleaner
Vinegar (*White Distilled*) – (*formula of ½ Distilled Vinegar
with ½ Water in a pump spray bottle*)

LAUNDRY DETERGENTS & SOAPS

All Free and Clear Liquid Laundry Detergent
Biofa Natural Wool Washing Liquid
Bi-O-Kleen Laundry Powder
Cal Ben Seafoam Laundry Soap
Dr. Bronner's Sal Suds (32 oz, $9.89 each)
Earth Rite Liquid Laundry Detergent
    (50 oz, case of 10 at $8.39 each)
Ecco Bella Laundry Powder/Liquid
Ecco Bella Suds Soap
Ecover Liquid Laundry Wash
    (53 oz, $8.69 each; 32 oz, $5.79 each)
Ecover Ultra Washing Powder (3 lb, $8.39 each)
Ecover Wool Wash Laundry Liquid (32 oz, $5.29)
Naturally Yours Laundry Detergent
Seventh Generation Laundry Liquid (32 oz, $6.49 each)
Seventh Generation Laundry Powder (48 oz, $6.99 each)
Simmons Pure Soaps (Vegetarian)
Sodasan Soap Washing Powder
Winter White Laundry Detergent Powder
Winter White Laundry Detergent Liquid
Woolite Cold Water Wash

LAUNDRY FABRIC SOFTENERS

For softening: Safe alternative for allergic or skin sensitive
individuals: Add ½ c. baking soda to the 1st rinse.

For softening & eliminating: Add ¼ c. distilled white vinegar
to the wash cycle.

Dryer Fresh
Ecover Fabric Softener (32 oz, case of 12 at $4.99 each)
Naturally Yours Natural Bleach and Softener
Shaklee Softer Than Soft Fabric conditioner

LAUNDRY SOIL & STAIN REMOVERS

All purpose stain remover: Mix ¼ c. borax with 2 c. cold water.
Soak total clothing article or soiled area only (works for blood,
chocolate, coffee, mildew and urine).

Bi-O-Kleen
Earth Wise
Naturally Yours All Purpose Spotter
Naturally Yours Enviro-Bright
Naturally Yours Natural Solvent Spotter

Metal Polishes

Hope's Brass Polish
Hope's Silver Polish
Kleen King Copper & Stainless Steel Cleaner Liquid
Parker's Perfect Polish Aluminum Stainless Steel
Weiman Royal Sterling Silver Polish

Oven Cleaners

The best strategy is to buy a self-cleaning oven.

Non-toxic overnight method: apply a small amount of baking soda to soiled areas. Let stand overnight. Then use a non-abrasive scouring pad to remove dirt. Rinse with water.

Microwaves should be clean with plain water only or a light dusting of baking soda on a sponge. Then rinse.

Ecover Cream Cleaner (32 oz, case of 12 at $5.09 each)

Scouring Powders

Arm & Hammer Baking Soda
  (*it is abrasive enough for tough stains and will deoderize and whiten*)
Borax
  (*formula: 1tsp. Borax; 2 T. distilled White Vinegar; 2 c. hot water in a refillable spray bottle*)
Ecover Cream Cleaner (32 oz, case of 12 at $5.09 each)
Granny's Old Fashioned Products Aloe Care

Toilet Bowl Cleaners

Earth Friendly Toilet Cleaner
  (16 oz, case of 12 at $3.29)
Earth Rite Toilet Bowl Cleaner
Ecover Toilet Cleaner
Sani-Flush Automatic Toilet Cleaner

REFERENCES

CHAPTER 1

American Academy of Allergy, Asthma and Immunology. 611 E. Wells Street, Milwaukee, WI 53202–3889. Phone: (414) 272-6071. *www.aaaai.org*

American Academy of Pediatrics. 141 Northwest Point Boulevard, Elk Grove Village, IL 60007-1098. Phone: (847) 434-4000. *www.aap.org*

Birdsall TC. "Gastrointestinal Candidiasis: Fact or fiction?" *Alternative Medicine Review*. 2(5):346–353, 1997.

Bircher AJ, et. al. "IgE to food allergens are highly prevalent in patients allergic to pollens, with and without symptoms of food allergy." *Clin Exp Allergy*. 24:367, 1997.

Bjarnason I, MacPherson A, Hollander D. "Intestinal permeability: An overview." *Gastroenterol*. 108:1566–1581, 1995.

Bodman FH. "The homeopathic treatment of allergic conditions." *British Homeopathic Journal*. (3), 1991.

Boris J and Mandel FS. "Foods and additives are common causes of attention deficit hyperactive disordern in children." *Ann Allergy*. May 1994, .

Braly J. *Food Allergy and Nutrition Revolution*. Connecticut: Keats Publishing. 1992.

Crook WG. "Can what a child eats make him dull, stupid, or hyperactive?" *Journal of Learning Disabilities*. 13:53–58, 1980.

Crook WG. *The Yeast Connection: A Medical Breakthrough*. 3rd ed. Jackson, Tennessee: Professional Books. 1986.

Feingold BF. *The Feingold Cookbook for Hyperactive Children and Others With Problems*. Random House. 1979.

Hilton E, Isenberg HD, Alperstein P, et. al. "Ingestion of yogurt containing Lactobacillus acidophilus asprophylaxis for candidal vaginitis." *Ann Intern Med*. 116:353–357, 1992.

Kennedy MJ, Voltz PA. "Ecology of Candida albicans gut colonization: Inhibition of Candida adhesion, colonization, and dissemination from the gastrointestinal tract by bacterial antagonism." *Infect Immun*. 49:654–663, 1985.

Kokkonen J, Ruuska T, Karttunen TJ, Niinimaki A. "Mucosal pathology of the foregut associated with food allergy and recurrent abdominal pains in children." *Acta Paediatr*. 90(1):16–21, Jan. 2001.

Kruzel T. *The Homeopathic Emergency Guide*. Berkley. California: North Atlantic Books. 1992.

Kumar V, Cotran RS, Robbins SL. *Basic Pathology*. 6th ed. Philadelphia, Pennsylvania: WB Saunders Co. 1997.

Lapidus CS, Schwarz DF, Honig PJ. "Atopic dermatitis in children: Who cares? Who pays?" *J Amer Acad Dermatology*. 28(5):699–703, 1993.

Leung DYM, Diaz LA, DeLeo V, Soter NA. "Allergic skin disorders and mastocytosis." *JAMA*. 278(22):1914–1923, 1997.

Linder MC. "Nutrition and metabolism of major minerals." *Nutritional Biochemistry and Metabolism with Clinical Applications*. 2nd ed. East Norwalk, Connecticut: Appleton & Lange. 1991.

Lipski E. *Digestive Wellness*. New Canaan, Connecticut: Keats Publishing, Inc. 1996.

Mahan LK and Escott-Stump L. *Krause's Food, Nutrition, & Diet Therapy*. 9th ed. Philadelphia: W.B. Saunders Co. 1996.

Marks D, Marks L. "Food Allergy: Manifestations, evaluation and management." *Postgraduate Medicine*. 93(2):191–201, February 1, 1993.

Marz RB. *Medical Nutrition from Marz*. 2nd ed. Portland, Oregon: Omni-Press. 1997.

Mitsuuoka T. "Intestinal Flora & Aging." *Nutrition Reviews*. 50(12): 438–46, Dec 1992.

Murray MT and Pizzorno JE. *Encyclopedia of Natural Medicine*. Rocklin, California: Prima Publishing.1991.

Pizzorno JE, Murray MT, eds. *Textbook of Natural Medicine*. 2nd ed. London: Churchill Livingstone. 1999.

Rapp DJ. *Is This Your Child? Discovering and Treating Unrecognized Allergies in Children and Adults*. New York: William Morrow & Co. 1991.

Ray NF, Baraniuk JN, Thamer M, et. al. "Healthcare expenditures for sinusitis in 1996: Contributions of asthma, rhinitis, and other airway disorders." *J Allergy Clin Immunol*. 103:408–514, 1999.

Sampson HA. "Food allergy: From biology toward therapy." *www.hosppract.com* McGraw-Hill Companies, 2001.

Sampson HA. "Food allergy. Part 1: Immunogenesis and clinical disorders." *J Allergy Clin Immunol*. 103:717, 1999.

Shils ME, Olson JA, Shike M, Ross AC, eds. *Modern Nutrition in Health and Disease*. 9th ed. Philadelphia, Pennsylvania: Lippincott Williams & Wilkins. 1999.

Smith LH. *Feed Your Body Right: Understanding Your Individual Body Chemistry for Proper Nutrition Without Guesswork*. M Evans & Co. 1995.

Smith LH. *How to Raise a Healthy Child: Medical & Nutritional Advice from America's Best-Loved Pediatrician*. M Evans & Co. 1996.

Steinman HA. "'Hidden' allergens in foods." *J Allergy Clin Immunol*. 98: 241, 1996.

Taylor JF. *Special Diets and Kids: How to Keep Your Child on Any Prescribed Diet*.

Thomas CL. ed. *Taber's Cyclopedic Medical Dictionary*. 17th ed. Philadelphia, Pennsylvania: FA Davis. 1993.

Tierney LM, McPhee SJ, Papadakis MA, eds. *Current Medical Diagnosis & Treatment*. New York, New York: Lange Medical Books/McGraw-Hill. 2000.

United States. Centers for Disease Control and Prevention. *CDC/HCHS Vital Health Statistics, Advanced Data: National Ambulatory Medical Care Summary, 1994*. Apr 1996.

United States. Environmental Protection Agency. *Asthma and Indoor Environments*. *www.epa.gov/iaq/asthma/triggers* Washington, DC, 2000.

Vermeulen F. *Concordant Materia Medica*. 2nd ed. The Netherlands: Emryss bv Publishers. 1997.

Wagner RD, Pierson C, Warner T, et. al. "Biotherapeutic effects of probiotic bacteria on candidiasis in immunodeficient mice. *Infect Immun* 65:4165–4172, 1997.

Wallace JM. "Nutritional modulation of gut-immune system interactions in autoimmunity." *International Journal of Integrative Medicine*. Jan/Feb 2(1):1822, 2000.

Weintraub S. *Allergies and Holistic Healing*. Pleasant Grove, Utah: Woodland Publishing. 1997.

Wright JV. Dr. *Wright's Book of Nutritional Therapy*. Emmaus, Pennsylvania: Rodale Press. 1979.

Zimmerman M. *The ADD Nutrition Solution: A Drug-Free Thirty Day Plan.* Owl Books. 1999.

CHAPTER 2

American Academy of Allergy, *Asthma & Immunology. www.aaaai.org*

American Lung Association. Epidemiology and Statistics Unit. "Trends in asthma." *Morbidity and Mortality.* Nov 1998.

Anonymous. "Quercetin:monograph." *Altern Med Rev.* 3:140-143, 1998.

Anderson R, Hay I, van Wyk HA, et. al. "Ascorbic acid in bronchial asthma." *S Afr Med J.* 63:649, 1983.

"ATS Update: Future directions for research on diseases of the lung." *American Journal of Respiratory and Critical Care Medicine.* 158:320–334, 1998.

Au DH, Lemaitre RN, Randell Curtis J, et. al. "The risk of myocardial infarction associated with inhaled beta-adrenoceptor agonists." *Am J Respir Crit Care Med.* 161:827–830, 2000.

Barnes PJ. "Drug therapy: inhaled glucocorticoids for asthma." *N Engl J Med.* 332:868–875, 1995.

Beausoleil JL, Weldon DP, McGeady SJ. "Beta2-agonist metered dose inhaler overuse: Psychological and demographic profiles." *Pediatrics.* 99:40–43, 1997.

Bernard A, Desreumeaux P, Huglo D, et. al. "Clinical aspects of allergic disease. Increased intestinal permeability in bronchial asthma." *J Allergy Clin Immunol.* 97:1173–1178, 1996.

Blaylock R. *Excitotoxins: The Taste That Kills.* Sante Fe, New Mexico: Health Press. 1994.

Broughton KS, Johnson CS, Pace BK, et. al. "Reduced asthma symptoms with n-3 fatty acid ingestion are related to 5-series leukotriene production." *Am J Clin Nutr.* 65:1011–7, 1997.

Buist AS, Vollmer WM. "Preventing deaths from asthma." *N Engl J Med.* 331:1584–1585, 1994.

Caffarelli C, Deriu FM, Terzi V, et al. "Gastrointestinal symptoms in patients with asthma." *Arch Dis Child.* 82:131–135, 2000.

Ciarallo L, Sauer A, Shannon M. "Clinical efficacy of intravenous magnesium in moderate to severe asthma: Results of a randomized, placebo-controlled trial." *Arch Pediatr Adolesc Med.* 148:69, 1994.

Ciarallo L, Sauer AH, Shannon MW. "Intravenous magnesium therapy for moderate to severe pediatric asthma: Results of a randomized, placebo-controlled trial." *J Pediatr.* 129:809, 1996.

Coles LS. "Quercetin: A Review of Clinical Applications." *Natural Medicine.* Jul 2000. *www.nat-med.com/edit.*

CollippP.J, Goldzier S, Weiss N, et. al. "Pyridoxine treatment of childhood bronchial asthma." *Ann Allergy.* 35:93, 1975.

Diette GB, Skinner EA, Nguyen TTH, et. al, "Comparison of quality of care by specialist and generalist physicians as usual source of asthma care for children." *Pediatrics.* 2108:432–437, 2001.

Dry J, Vincent D. "Effect of a fish oil diet on asthma: results of a 1-year double-blind study." *Int Arch Allergy Appl Immunol.* 95:156–7, 1991.

Eaton T, Withy S, Garrett JE, et. al. "Spirometry in primary care practice: the importance of quality assurance and the impact of spirometry workshops. *Chest.* Aug 116(2):416–423, 1999.

Farooqi IS, Hopkin JM. "Early childhood infection and atopic disorder." *Thorax.* Nov 53:927–932, 1998.

Fauci AS, Braunwald E, Isselbacher KJ, et. al. *Harrison's Principles of Internal Medicine Companion Handbook.* 14th ed., New York: McGraw-Hill. 1998. p. 722.

Fogarty A, Britton J. "The role of diet in the aetiology of asthma." *Clin Exp Allergy*. 30:615–27, 2000.

Fogarty A, Lewis S, Weiss S, Britton J. "Dietary vitamin E, IgE concentrations, and atopy." *Lancet*. 356(9241):1573–4, Nov 4, 2000.

Hardman JG, Limbird LE. eds. Goodman & Gilman's *The Pharmacological Basis of Therapeutics*. 9th ed. New York: McGraw-Hill. 1996.

Hill J, Micklewright A, Lewis, Britton J. "Investigation of the effect of short-term change in dietary magnesium intake in asthma." *Eur Respir J*. 10:2225–9, 1997.

Hijazi N, Abalkhail B, Seaton A. "Diet and childhood asthma in a society in transition: a study in urban and rural Saudi Arabia." *Thorax*. 55:775–779, Sep 2000.

Hodge L, Salome CM, Hughes, et. al. "Effects of dietary intake of omega-3 and omega-6 fatty acids on severity of asthma in children." *Eur Respir J*. 11:361–5, 1997.

Hodge L, Salome CM, Peat JK, et. al. "Consumption of oily fish and child-hood asthma risk." *Med J Austral*. 164:137–40, 1996.

Husby S. "Sensitization and tolerance." *Allergy Clin Immuno*. 1(3) :237–241, Jun 2001.

Juntti H, Tikkanen S, KokkonenJ, et. al. "Cow's milk allergy is associated with recurrent otitis media during childhood." *Acta Otolaryngol*. 119(8):867–73, 1999.

Kelly GS. "Hydrochloric acid: physiological functions and clinical implications." *Altern Med Rev*. 2:116–127, 1997.

Kemp T, Pearce N, Fitharris P, et. al. "Is infant immunization a risk factor for childhood asthma or allergy?" *Epidemiology*. 8:678–680, 1997.

Kirsch CM, Payan DG, Wong MY, et. al. "Effect of eicosapentaenoic acid in asthma." *Clin Allergy*. 18:177–87, 1988.

Kokkonen J, Ruuska T, Karttunen TJ, Niinimaki A. "Mucosal pathology of the foregut associated with food allergy and recurrent abdominal pains in children." *Acta Paediatr*. 90(1):16–21, Jan 2001.

Kokkonen J, Simila S, Herva R. "Impaired gastric function in children with cow's milk intolerance." *Eur J Pediatr*. 132(1):1–6, Sep 1979.

Kokkonen J, Tikkanen, Savilahti E. "Residual intestinal disease after milk allergy in infancy." *J Pediatr Gastroenterol Nutr*. 32(2):156–61, Feb 2001.

Kumar V, Contran RS, Robbins SL. *Basic Pathology*. 6th ed. Philadelphia: W.B. Saunders Company. 1997.

LeGros G, Erb K, Harris N, et. al. "Immunoregulatory networks in asthma." *Clin Exp Allergy*. 28:S92–96, 1998.

Lemanske RF, Allen DB. "Choosing a long-term controller medication in childhood asthma. The proverbial two-edged sword." *Am J Respir Crit Care Med*. 156:988–991, 1997.

Li X, Ward C, Thien F., et. al. "An antiinflammatory effect of salmeterol, a long-acting beta2 agonist, assessed in airway biopsies and bronchoalveo-lar lavage in asthma." *Am J Respir Crit Care Med*. 160: 1493–1499, 1999.

Mancuso CA, Peterson MG, Charlson ME. "Effects of depressive symptoms on health-related quality of life in asthma patients." *J Gen Intern Med*. 15:301–310, 2000.

Mansfield LE, Stein MR. "Gastroesophageal reflux and asthma: a possible reflux mechanism." *Ann Allergy*. 41:224-226, 1978.

Marz RB. *Medical Nutrition from Marz*. 2nd ed. Portland, Oregon: Omni-Press. 1997.

McFadden ER. "Improper patient techniques and metered dose inhalers: Clinical consequences and solutions to misuse." *J Allergy Clin Immunol*. 96:278, 1995.

Meier CR, Jick H. "Drug use and pulmonary death rates in increasingly symptomatic asthma patients in the UK." *Thorax*. 52(7):612–617, Jul 1997.

Miller AL. "The etiologies, pathophysiology, and alternative/complementary treatment of asthma." *Altern Med Rev*. 6(1):20–47, 2001.

Morild I, Giertsen JC. "Sudden death from asthma." *Forensic Sci Int*. 42(1–2):145–50, Jul 1989.

Murray MT. "Natural relief for asthma and hay fever." *Health Counselor*. 4(3):30–33, 1999.

Murray MT. *Encyclopedia of Nutritional Supplements*. Rocklin, California: Prima Publishing. 1996.

Nagakura T, Matsuda S, Shichijyo K, et. al. "Dietary supplementation with fish oil rich in omega-3 polyunsaturated fatty acids in children with bronchial asthma." *Eur Respir J*. 16:861–865, 2000.

National Asthma Education and Prevention Program. *Expert Panel Report II: Guidelines for the Diagnosis and Management of Asthma*. Bethesda, Maryland: U.S. Department of Health and Human Services Publication No. 97–4051, 1997.

Nekam KL. "Nutritional triggers in asthma." *Acta Microbio Immunol Hung*. 45:113–117, 1998.

Nelson HS. "Drug therapy: beta-adrenergic bronchodilators." *N Engl J Med*. 333:499–507, Aug 24, 1995.

O'Byrne PM, Kerstjens HAM. "Inhaled beta2-agonists in the treatment of asthma." *N Engl J Med*. 335:886–888, 1996.

Pabon H, Monem G, Kissoon N. "Safety and efficacy of magnesium sulfate infusions in children with status asthmaticus." *Ped Emerg Care*. 10:200, 1994.

Parronchi P, Brugnolo F, Sampognaro S, Maggi E. "Genetic and environmental factors contributing to the onset of allergic disorders." *Int Arch Allergy Immunol*. 121:2–9, 2000.

Pearce F, Befus AD, Bienenstock J. "Mucosal mast cells, III, Effect of quercetin and other flavonoids on antigen-induced histamine secretion from rat intestinal mast cells." *J Allergy Clin Immunol*. 73:819–823, 1984.

Powell CVE, Nash AA, Powers HJ, Primhak RA. "Antioxidant status in asthma." *Ped Pulmonology*. 18:34–38, 1994.

Rea HH, Garrett JE, Lanes SF, et.al. "The association between asthma drugs and severe life-threatening attacks." *Chest*. 110(6):1446–51, Dec 1996.

Richter JE. "Gastroesophageal reflux disease and asthma: the two are directly related." *Am J Med*. 108:153S–158S, 2000.

Ritz T, Steptoe A, DeWilde S, Costa M. "Emotions and stress increase respiratory resistance in asthma." *Psychosom Med*. 62:401–412, 2000.

Schwartz J. "Dietary factors and their relation to respiratory symptoms." *Am J Epid*. 132:67, 1990.

Schwartz J, Weiss ST. "Relationship between dietary vitamin C intake and pulmonary function in the first national health and nutrition examination survey (NHANES 1)." *Am J Clin Nutr*. 59:110–114, 1994.

Schwartz, MW, Curry TA, Sargent AJ, Blum NJ, Fein JA. *Pediatric Primary Care: A Problem-Oriented Approach*. 3rd ed. St. Louis, Missouri: Mosby-Year Book, Inc. 1997.

Shanmugasundaram KR, Kumar SS, Rajajee S. "Excessive free radical generation in the blood of children suffering from asthma." *Clin Chim Acta*. 305(1-2):107–14, Mar 2001.

Singh V, Jain NK. "Asthma as a cause for, rather than a result of, gastroesophageal reflux." *J Asthma*. 20:241–243, 1983.

Skobeloff EM, et. al. "Intravenous magnesium sulfate for the treatment of acute asthma in the emergency department." *JAMA*. 262:1210–1213, 1989.

Sontag S. "Why do the published data fail to clarify the relationship between gastroesophageal reflux and asthma?" *Am J Med.* 108:159S–169S, 2000.

Spitzer WO, Suissa S, Ernst P, et. al. "The use of beta-agonists and the risk of death and near death from asthma." *N Engl J Med.* 326:501–506, Feb 20,1992.

Suissa S, Ernst P, Benayoun S, et. al. "Low-dose inhaled corticosteroids and the prevention of death from asthma." *N Engl J Med.* 343:332–336, Aug 3, 2000.

Suissa S, Ernst P, Zahger D, et. al. "Albuterol in mild asthma." *N Engl J Med.* 336:729–730, 1997.

Tierney LM, McPhee SJ, Papadakis MA. eds. *Current Medical Diagnosis & Treatment.* 39th ed. New York: Lange Medical Books/McGraw-Hill. 2000.

Tikkanen S, Kokkonen J, Juntti H, Niinimaki A. "Status of children with cow's milk allergy in infancy by 10 years of age." *Acta Paediatr.* 89(10):1174–80, Oct 2000.

Trenga CA, Koenig JQ, Williams PV. "Dietary antioxidants and ozone-induced bronchial hyperresponsiveness in adults with asthma." *Arch Environ Health.* 56(3):242-9, May–Jun 2001.

Turner MO, Noertjojo K, Vedal S. "Risk factors for near-fatal asthma. A case-controlled study in hospitalized patients with asthma." *Am J Respir Crit Care Med.* 157:1804–1809, 1997.

United States. Centers for Disease Control. "Forecasted state-specific estimates of self-reported asthma prevalence-1998." *Morbidity and Mortality.* 47:1022–1025, Dec. 4, 1998.

United States. Environmental Protection Agency. Asthma and Indoor Environments. Washington, DC. Available at: *http://www.epa.gov/iaq/asthma/index.html*

United States. National Institute of Allergy and Infectious Disease. *Asthma: A concern for minority populations.* Jan 1997.

Vural H, Uzun K. "Serum and red blood cell antioxidant status in patients with bronchial asthma. *Can Respir J.* 7(6):476–480, Nov 2000.

Werner HA. "Status asthmaticus in children: A review." *Chest.* 119: 1913–1929, 2001.

Wickens K, Pearce N, Crane J, Beasley R. "Antibiotic use in early childhood and the development of asthma." *Clin Exp Allergy.* 29:766–771, 1999.

Wright JV. Childhood Asthma. 1(3), July 2001. Available from *www.jvwonline.com* or Publishers Management Group 800-528-0559.

Wright JV. "Treatment of childhood asthma with parenteral vitamin B_{12}, gastric reacidification, and attention to food allergy, magnesium, and pyridoxine. Three case reports with background and an integrated hypothesis." *J Nutr Med.* 1:277–282, 1990.

Zand, J, Walton R, Rountree, B. *Smart Medicine for a Healthier Child.* Garden City, New York: Avery Publishing Group. 1994.

CHAPTER 3

Adams PF and Marano MA. "Current estimates from the National Health Interview Survey, 1994." National Center for Health Statistics. *Vital Health Stat.* 10(193), 1995.

Albertson AM, Tobelman RO, Engstrom A, et. al. "Nutrient intakes of 2–10 year old American children: 10 year trends." *Journal of the American Dietetic Association.* 92:142-6, 1992.

Beisel WR. "Single nutrients and immunity." *American Journal of Clinical Nutrition.* 35(Suppl.):417, 1982.

Beisel WR, et. al. "Single-nutrient effects on immunological functions." *JAMA.* 245(1):53, Jan. 2, 1981.

Beisel WR. "The history of nutritional immunology." *Journal of Nutritional Immunology.* 1(1):5, 1992.

Birch LL, Johnston SL, Fisher JA. "Children's eating: the development of food acceptance patterns." *Young Children.* 50:71–78, 1995.

Birch LL, Marlin DW. "I don't like it; I never tried it: effects of exposure on two-year-old children's food preferences." *Appetite.* 3:353–360, 1982.

Bower RH. "Nutrition and immune function." *Nutrition in Clinical Practice.* 5(5):189, 1990.

Bronk I, Gober AE. "Prophalaxis with amoxicillin or sulfisoxazole for OM: effect on the recovery of penicillin-resistant bacteria from children. *Clin Infect Dis.* 42:353–56, 1996.

Bender BS. "Barbara, What's a Nice Girl Like You Doing Writing an Article Like This? The Scientific Basis of Folk Remedies for Colds and Flu." *Chest.* 118:887–888, 2000.

Butler JC, Hofmann J, et. al. "The continued emergence of drug-resistant Streptococcus pneumoniae in the United States: An update from the CDC's Pneumococcal Sentinel Surveillance System. *J Infect Dis.* 174:986–93, 1996.

Cerra FB. "Immune system modulation: Nutritional and pharmacologic approaches." *Critical Care Medicine.* 18(2), Jan 1990.

Cerra FB. "Nutrient modulation of inflammatory and immune function." *American Journal of Surgery.* 161:230, Feb 1991.

Dagan W, Abramson O, et. al. "Impaired bacteriologic response to oral cephalosporins in acute otitis media caused by pneumococci with intermediate resistance to penicillin." *Pediatr Infect Dis J.* 15:980–85, 1986.

Dowell SF, Schwartz B. "Resistance pneumococci: Protecting patients through judicious antibiotic use." *Am Fam Physician.* 55:1647–54, 1997.

Dowell SH, Marcy SM, Phillips WR, et. al. "Principles of judicious use of antimicrobial agents for pediatric upper respiratory tract infections." *Pediatrics.* 101:163–165, 1998.

Garre MA, et. al. "Current concepts in immune derangement due to undernutrition." *Journal of Parenteral and Enteral Nutrition.* 11(3):309, 1987.

Haas, EM. *Staying Healthy with the Seasons.* Berkeley, California: Celestial Arts. 1981.

Helstrom PB, Balish E. "Effect of oral tetracycline, the microbial flora, and the athymic state on gastrointestinal colonization and infection of BA1B/c mice with candida albicans." *Infection and Immunity.* pp. 764–74, Mar 1979.

Ilback NG. "Effects of methyl mercury exposure on spleen and blood natural killer (NK) cell activity in the mouse." *Toxicology.* 25(1):117, Mar 1991.

Jones CLA. *The Antibiotic Alternative: The Natural Guide to Fighting Infection and Maintaining a Healthy Immune System.* Healing Arts Press. 2000.

Katzung BG. ed. *Basic & Clinical Pharmacology.* Norwalk, Connecticut: Appleton & Lange. 1995.

Lavine JB. "Chicken Soup or Jewish Medicine ." *Chest.* 119:1295, 2001.

Lieberman MD. "Effects of nutrient substrates on immune function." *Nutrition.* 6(1):88, 1990.

McCaig L, Hughes J. "Trends in antimicrobial drug prescribing among office-based physicians in the United States." *JAMA.* 273:214–219, 1995.

National Institute of Allergy and Infectious Diseases. *Is It a Cold or the Flu?* Apr 2001.

Nord CE, Edlund C. "Impact of antimicrobial agents on human intestinal microflora." *J. Chemotherapy.* 2(4):218–37, 1990.

Ohry A, Tsafrir J. "Is chicken soup an essential drug?" *CMAJ.* 162(7):973, Apr. 2000.

Pitchford P. *Healing with Whole Foods: Oriental Traditions and Modern Nutrition.* Berkeley, California: North Atlantic Books. 1993.

Quillin P, Quillin N. *Beating Cancer with Nutrition.* Tulsa: Nutrition Times Press. 2001.

Rennard BO, Ertl RF, Gossman GL, Robbins RA, Rennard SI. "Chicken Soup Inhibits Neutrophil Chemotaxis In Vitro." *Chest.* 118:1150–1157, 2000.

Rosner F. "Therapeutic efficacy of chicken soup." *Chest.* 78:672–674, 1980.

Saketkhoo K, Januszkiewicz A, Sackner MA. "Effects of drinking hot water, cold water, and chicken soup on nasal mucus velocity and nasal airflow resistance." *Chest.* 74:408–410, 1978.

Schmidt MA, Smith LH, Sehnert KW. *Beyond Antibiotics: 50 (or so) Ways to Boost Immunity and Avoid Antibiotics.* Berkeley, California: North Atlantic Books. 1994.

Schmidt MA. *Healing Childhood Ear Infections: Prevention, Home Care, and Alternative Treatment.* Berkeley, California: North Atlantic Books. 1996.

Schwitters B, Masquerlier J. *OPC in Practice: Biflavanols and their application.* Rome: Alfa Omega. 1993.

Welch HG. "Antibiotic resistance: A new kind of epidemic." *Postgraduate Medicine.* 76(6):Nov 1, 1984.

CHAPTER 4

Allman, William F. "Aspartame: Some Bitter with the Sweet?" *Science.* vol. 5, July/August, 1984, p. 14.

Arnold, L.E. et al. "Megavitamins for minimal brain dysfunction: A placebo-controlled study." *JAMA.* 240:2642, 1978.

Association for Applied Psychophysiology and Biofeedback. "What Kinds of Problems can Biofeedback Help? What is Biofeedback?" *http://www.aapb.org/public/articles/details.cfm?id=7*

Atkins, Robert M.D. "Hyperactivity's True Tragedy." *Health Revelations.* Vol. IV, No. 9, September 1996.

Balch, James F., & Balch, Phyllis A. *Prescription for Nutritional Healing.* Garden City Park, NY: Avery Publishing Group, 1997, pp. 148–9, 330–3.

Barkley, R., Cunningham, C. "Do stimulant drugs improve the academic performance of hyperkinetic children." *Clinical Pediatrics.* 1978, vol. 17, pp. 85–92.

Barkley, R. "A review of stimulant drug research with hyperactive children." *Journal of Child Psychology and Psychiatry.* 1977, vol. 18, pp. 137–165.

Barkley, R., Ullman, D. "A comparison of objective measures of activity and distractibility in hyperactive and non hyperactive children." *Journal of Abnormal Psychology.* vol. 3, pp. 231–244, 1975.

Barlow, PJ. "A pilot study of metal levels in the hair of hyperactive children." *Med Hypotheses.* 11(3):309–18, 1983.

Bekaroglu, M. et al. "Relationships between serum free fatty acids and zinc, and attention deficit hyperactivity disorder: a research note. *J Child Psychol Psychiatry.* 37(2):225–7, 1996.

Benson H, Shapiro D, Tursky B, Schwartz GE. "Decreased Systolic Blood Pressure Through Operant Conditioning Techniques in Patients with Essential Hypertension." *Science.* 217, 1971.

Benton, David & Roberts, Gwilym. "Effect of vitamin and mineral supplementation on intelligence of a sample of school children." *The Lancet.* January 23, pp. 140–143, 1988.

Benton, D. "Dietary sugar, hyperactivity, and cognitive functioning: a methodological review." *J. Appl Nutr.* 41(1): 13–22, 1989.

Benton, D. "Vitamin and mineral intake and cognitive function," in A. Bendich, CE Butterworth (Eds.), *Micronutrients in Health and Disease.* New York: Marcel Dekker, 1991.

Black, Dean. "Diet and Behavior." *The Healing Currents Series.* Springville, UT: Tapestry Press, 1989.

Boris, M. & Mandel, F. "Foods and additives are common causes of the attention deficit hyperactive disorder in children." *Annals of Allergy.* 72(5): 462–7, 1993.

Bosco, J., Robin, S. *Hyperkinesis: prevalence and treatment.* New York Academic Press: 1980, p. 173.

Boyages, SC et al. "Iodine deficiency impairs intellectual and neuromotor development inapparently-normal persons." A study of rural inhabitants of northcentral China. *Med J Aust.* 150(12):676–82, 1989.

Brenner, A. "The effects of megadoses of selected B-complex vitamins on children with hyperkinesis: controlled studies with long-term follow-up." *Journal of Learning Disabilities.* vol. 15, 258–264, May 1982.

Brin, M. "Behavioral effects of energy and protein deficits." DHEW (NIH) publication no. 79–1966, Washington DC: Department of Health, Education and Welfare, 1973.

Brocksmith, Carolyn Gallagher. "New diet can eliminate attention deficit disorder." *Opinion.* August 26, 1999.

Bruce, Gene. "Fighting Mandatory Ritalin in the Schools." *East West.* pp. 39–44, December 1988.

Budzynski T & Stoyva J. "An Instrument for Producing Deep Muscle Relaxation by Means of Analog Information Feedback." *Journal of Applied Behavioral Analysis.* 2:231–237, 1969.

Buist, Robert. *Food Chemical Sensitivity.* Garden City Park, NY: Avery Publishing Group, Inc., 1988.

Campbell, Bill. "Control Hyperactivity Naturally." *Better Nutrition.* June 1989, pp. 14, 30.

Cantwell, D. "A critical review of therapeutic modalities with hyperactive children." New York: Spectrum Publications, 1975.

Cantwell, D. "Genetic studies of hyperkinetic children." *Genetic Research in Psychiatry.* John Hopkins University Press, 1975.

Cantwell, D. "Hyperkinetic Syndrome." *Child Psychiatry.* Oxford. pp. 524–555, 1975.

Collip, PJ. Et al. "Manganese in infant formulas and learning disability. *Ann Nutr Metab.* 27:488–494, 1983.

Colquhoun I, Bunday S. "A lack of essential fatty acids as a possible cause of hyperactivity in children." *Med. Hypotheses.* 7: 673–9, 1981.

Condemi, John J. "Aspirin and Food Dye Reactions." *Bulletin of the New York Academy of Medicine.* Vol. 57, pp. 600–607, September 1981.

Conners, C.K. *Feeding the Brain.* New York: Plenum Press, 1989.

Conners, C.K. *Food Additives and Hyperactive Children.* New York: Plenum Press, 1980, pp. 107, 110.

Cowley, Geoffrey. "The Not-Young and the Restless." *Newsweek.* July 26, 1993; pp. 48–49.

Crawford, MJ. "The role of essential fatty acids in neural development: implications for perinatal nutrition." *American Journal of Clinical Nutrition.* 1993; 57(suppl.): 703S–10S.

Crook, WG. Nutrition, food allergies, and environmental toxins. *Letter. J Learn Disabil.* 20(5):260–261, 1987.

Crook, William G. *Help for the Hyperactive Child.* Professional Books, 1991.

Crook, William G. *Solving the Puzzle of Your Hard To Raise Child.*

Crook, William G. *Yeast, ADHD and Ear Infections.*

Curtin, Jean. "Autism and Allergies? One little boy's story." *Pure Facts Newsletter of the Feingold Associations of the United States.* Dec 1995/Jan 1996, Vol. 19, No. 10.

David, O. et al. "Lead and hyperactivity." *Lancet.* 2:900–3, 1972.

Dean, Ward. "Are Doctors Sugar-Coating Attention Deficit Diagnoses?" *Nutritional News Newsletter of Vitamin Research Products, Inc.* August 1997, Vol. 11, No.8.

de Deckere, E.A., et al. "Health Aspects of fish and n-3 polyunsaturated fatty acids from plant and marine origin." *Eur J Clin Nutr.* 52(10):749–53, 1998.

De Lorgeril, M., et al. "Mediterranean alpha-linoleic acid-rich diet in secondary prevention of coronary heart disease." *Lancet.* 343:1454–1459, 1994.

Dudek, B. and D. Merecz. "Impairment of psychological functions in children environmentally exposed to lead. *Int J Occup Med Environ Health.* 10(1):37–46, 1997.

Eck, P. "Vitamins and Minerals." *Healthview Newsletter.* 1981, Nos. 27–29.

Eck, Paul & Wilson, Larry. "Insights into Learning Disorders and Hyperactivity." *The Nutrition and Dietary Consultant.* Feb 1988, pp. 9, 14.

Egger, Joseph. "The Hyperkinetic Syndrome." Food Allergy and Intolerance, London: Medical Press, pp. 674–686, 1987.

Egger, J., Carter CM. "A dietary management of severe childhood migraine." *Nutrition, Applied Nutrition.* 39A: pp. 294–303, 1985.

Egger, J. et al. "Controlled trial of oligoantigenic treatment in the hyperkinetic syndrome." *Lancet.* 1:540–5, 1985.

Erkfritz, Dr. Gary. *AD/HD Update.* Volume I, Issue 3. June–July 2000.

Feingold, BF. "Hyperkinesis and learning disabilities linked to ingestion of artificial food colors and flavors. *J Learn Disabil.* 9(9):551–9, 1976.

Feingold, Ben F. *Why Your Child is Hyperactive.* New York: Random House, 1985.

Feingold, Helene, & Feingold, Ben. *The Feingold Cookbook for Hyperactive Children and Others with Problems Associated with Food Additives and Salicylates.* New York: Random House, 1979.

Firestone, P. et al. "The effects of caffeine on hyperactive children." *J Learn Disabil.* 11(3):133–141, 1978.

Fisher, Marjorie. "Foods and Chemicals Can Make Children Ill." *NOHA News.* Fall 1992. Vol. XVII, No. 4.

Fisher, Marjorie. "Attention Deficit Hyperactivity Disorder (ADHD)" *NOHA News.* Winter 2000. Vol. XXV, No. 1.

Garrett BL & Silver MP. "The Use of EMG and Alpha Biofeedback to Relieve Test Anxiety in College Students." Read before the American Psychological Association meeting, Washington D.C.,1972.

Gibson, RA. "The effect of dietary supplementation with evening primrose oil on hyperkinetic children." *Proc Nutr Soc Aust.* 10:196, 1985.

Gittelman, R., Eskenazi, B. "Lead and hyperactivity revisited. An investigation of Nondisadvantaged children." *Arch. Gen. Psychol.* 1986; 14:565–77.

Goldman, JA. Et al. "Behavioral effects of sucrose on preschool childen." *J Abnorm Child Psychol.* 14(4):656–77, 1986.

Goodwin, D.W. et al. "Alcoholism and the Hyperactive Child Syndrome." *J Nerv.Ment. Dis.* 160; 349–53, 1975.

Gordon, S. "Junk food linked to low test scores." *The Modesto Bee* (California), November 16, 1986, p. 1.

Gorman PJ & Kamiya J. "Operant Conditioning of Stomach Acid pH." Read before the Biofeedback Research Society Meeting, Boston. 1972.

Gross, M.D. "Effect of sucrose on hyperkinetic children." *Pediatrics.* 74(5): 876–7, 1984.

Haley, J.P., Ray, R.S., Tomasi, L. et al. "Hyperkinesis and food additives: testing the Feingold hypothesis." *Pediatrics*. 61:818–28, 1978.

Hardych DC, Petrinovich LF, Ellsworth DW. "Feedback of Speech Muscle Activity During Silent Reading: Two Comments. *Science*. 157:581, 1967.

Harrell, R.F. "Further effects of added thiamin on learning and, other processes." New York: Teachers College, Columbia University, 1947.

Haslam, R.H.A. et al. "Effects of megavitamin therapy on children with attention deficit disorders." *Pediatrics*. 74:103–111, 1984.Heeley, A.G., and Roberts, G.E. "A study of triptophan metabolism in psychotic children." *Developmental Medicine and Child Neurology*. 3, 708–718, 1966.

Hesser, Lynn. "Tartrazine on Trial." *Food and Chemical Toxicology*. Vol. 22, pp. 1019–1024, Dec 1984.

Hill, GM "The impact of breakfast especially ready-to-eat cereals on nutrient intake and health of children." *Nutr Res*. 15(4):595–613, 1995.

Hoffer, A. "Treatment of hyperkinetic children with nicotinamide and pyridoxine." Letter to the editor. *Can. Med. Assoc. J*. 107:111–12, 1972.

Hoffer, A. "Vitamin B_3 dependent child." *Schizophrenia*. 3:107–113, 1971.

Hole, K. et al. "Lead intoxication as an etiologic factor in hyperkinetic behavior in children." *Acta Paediatr. Scand*. 68:759, 1979.

Holmes, L. "Biofeedback". *Mental Health Resources*. 9/20/99. *http://mentalhealth.about.com/library/weekly/aa092099.htm*

Howard, JMH. "Clinical import of small increases in serum aluminum." *Clin Chem*. 30(10): 1722–3, 1984.

Hunter, Beatrice Trum. *Consumer Beware!* New York: Charles Scribner's and Sons, 1976.

Hunter, Beatrice Trum. *The Great Nutrition Robbery*. New York: Charles Scribner's and Sons, 1978.

Hyperkinesis (Overactivity in Children). Pueblo, CO: Systems DC, 1981.

Irwin M. et al. "Tryptophan metabolism in children with attention deficit disorder. *Am J Psychiatry*. 138(8):1082–5, 1981.

Jacobson, MF. "Effects of sugar on behavior in children." Letter. *JAMA*. 275(10): 756–7, 1996.

Kozielec, T. et al. "Deficiency of certain trace elements in children with hyperactivity." *Psychiatr Pol*. 28(3):345–53, 1994 (in Polish).

Kozielec, T. and B. Starobrat-Hermelin. "Assessment of magnesium levels in children with attention deficit hyperactivity disorder (ADHD)." *Magnes Res*. 10(2):143–8, 1997.

LeFever, Gretchen, Dawson, Keila V., Morrow, Ardythe L. "The Extent of Drug Therapy for Attention Deficit Disorder Among Children in Public Schools." *American Journal of Public Health*. September 1999, Vol.89, No.9., pp. 1359–1364."

LeRiche, W. Harding. *A Chemical Feast*. New York: Facts on File Publications, 1982.

Lesser, M. *Nutrition and Vitamin Therapy*. New York: Bantam Books, 1980.

Lester ML et al. "Refined carbohydrate intake, hair cadmium levels and cognitive functioning in children." *Nutr Behav*. 1:3–13, 1982.

Liebman, Bonnie. " The All-American Junk Food Diet." *Nutrition Action Newsletter*. May 1988, p. 8.

Magu, Joseph A., Tu, Anthony T. *Food Additive Toxicology*. New York: Marcel Dekker, Inc., 1995.

Mahan, K et al., "Sugar Allergy and Childrens' Behavior. *Abstract. Immunology and Allergy Practice*, p. 81, July 1985.

Maher, Timothy J. "Neurotoxicology of Food Additives." *Neurotoxicology*. v. 7, pp. 183–196, Summer 1986

Malter, R. "Implications of bio-nutritional approach to the diagnosis, treatment, and cost of learning disabilities." Paper presented at the Association for Children with Learning Disabilities International Conference, Washington D.C., 1983.

McGee, Charles. *How to Survive Modern Technology.* New Cannan: Keats, 1979.

Messina, Virginia. "Is NutraSweet Safe?" *Pure Facts Newsletter of the Feingold Associations of the United States.* Vol. 14, No. 3, April 1990

Milich, R., Wolraich, M, Lindgren, S. "Sugar and hyperactivity: a critical review of empirical findings." *Clin Psychol Rev.* 6:493–513, 1986.

Mindell, Earl. *Unsafe at Any Meal.* New York: Warner Books, 1987.

Moses, Susan. "Food Coloring May Alter Kids' Behavior." *The APA Monitor.* October 1989.

Mu-oz, KA, et al. "Food intakes of U.S. children and adolescents compared with recommendations." *Pediatrics.* 100(3):323–9, 1997 Sep.

Nelson, M. "Workshop on 'nutrition and the school child' – food, vitamins and IQ." *Proc Nutr Soc.* 50:29c35, 1991.

Nemzer, ED. Et al. Amino acid supplementation as therapy for attention deficit disorder." *J Am Acad Child Psychiatry.* 25:509–13, 1986.

O'Hair, DE. "Biofeedback: Review, History and Application." *http://www.users.cts.com/crash/d/deohair/psyhoph.html*

Olney, John W. "Excitatory neurotoxins as Food Additives: An Evaluation of Risk." *Neurotoxicology.* v. 2, January 1981, pp. 163–192.

Perara, Judth. "Authorities Ban Food Coloring from School Dinners." *New Scientist.* v. 111, 8/14/86, p. 14.

Pfeiffer, C. *Mental and Elemental Nutrients: A Guide to Nutrition and Health Care.* New Canaan: Keats, 1975.

Pihl, R. & Parkes, M. "Hair element content in LD children." *Science.* pp. 204–6, 1977.

Prinz, R.J. et al. "Dietary correlates of hyperactive behavior in children." *J. Consulting Clin. Psychol.* 48: 760–9, 1980.

"Pure Facts" Newsletter of the Feingold Associations of the United States. (ongoing newsletter with specific references to salicytate-free diets of autism, ADD, ADHD, and Learning disabilities.)

Raiten, DJ et al. "Vitamin and trace element assessment of autistic and learning disabled children." *Nutr Behav.* 2:9–17, 1994.

Rapp, Doris J. *Allergies and the Hyperactive Child.* New York: Sovereign Books, 1979.

Reichenberg-Ullman, Judyth. "Homeopathy for Hyperactive Children." *Natural Health.* pp. 70–73, 106–107, Nov/Dec 1992.

Rimland, B. & Larson, G. "Hair mineral analysis and behavior: analysys of 51 studies." *Journal of Learning Disabilities.* v. 16, pp. 279–285, May 1983.

Robbins, John. "Recess for Ritalin." *Natural Health.* pp. 60–63, March–April 1997.

Rowe, Katherine & Rowe, Kenneth. "Synthetic food coloring and behavior, a dose response effect in a double-blind, placebo-controlled, repeated measures study." *J Pediatrics.* 1994; 125:691: 8.

Sadler, M.J. "Recent Aspartame Studies." *Food and Chemical Toxicology.* v. 22, 9/84, pp. 771–773.

Salamy, J. et al. "Physiological Changes in Hyperactive Children Following the Ingestion of Food Additives." *International Journal of Neuroscience.* Vol 16, pp. 241–246, May 1982.

Sargent JD, Green EE, Walters ED. "The Autogenic Feedback Training in a Pilot Study of Migraine and Tension Headaches." *Headache.* 12:120–125, 1972.

Schecter, MD, Gibbons, GD. "Objectively measured hyperactivity. II. Caffeine and amphetamine effects." *J Clin Pharmacol.* 25:276–80, 1985.

Schmidt, M.A. *Smart Fats: How Dietary Fats and Oils Affect Mental, Physical and Emotional Intelligence.* Frog, Ltd., 1997.

Schmidt, M.H. et al. "Does oligoantigenic diet influence hyperactive/ conduct-disordered children – a controlled trial." *Eur Child Adolesc Psychiatry.* 6(2):88–95, 1997.

Schoeder, HA. "Losses of vitamins and trace minerals resulting from processing and preservation of foods." *Am J Clin Nutr.* 24:562–73, 1971.

Schoenthaler, Stephen J. "Sugar and children's behavior." *The New England Journal of Medicine.* June 30, 1994, Vol. 330, No. 26, pp. 1901–4.

Schoenthaler, Stephen J., Walter E. Doraz, and James A. Wakefield, Jr. "The Impact of a Low Food Additive and Sucrose Diet on Academic Performance in 803 New York City Public Schools." *Int. J. Biosocial Research.* 8(2):185–195, 1986.

Schoenthaler, Stephen J., Walter E. Doraz, and James A. Wakefield, Jr. "The Testing of Various Hypotheses as Explanations for the Gains in National Standardized Academic Test Scores in the 1978–1983 New York City Nutrition Policy Modification Project." *Int. J Biosocial Research.* Vol. 8(2): 196–203, 1986.

Sever, Y. et al. "Iron treatment in children with attention deficit hyperactivity disorder." *Neuropsychobiology.* 35: 178–80, 1997.

Sodhi, Virender. "Treating Attention Deficit Disorder the Ayurvedic Way." *Health Supplement Retailer.* pp. 42–43, October 1997.

South, J. "Natural Remedies for ADD." *Nutritional News.* 11(9), September 1997.

Spring, B. & Wurtman, RJ. "Effects of food and nutrients on the behavior of normal individuals." In: Wurtman JJ, editor. *Nutrition and the Brain.* Volume 7. New York: Raven Press; p. 1–47, 1985.

Starobrat-Hermelin B. and T. Kozielec. "The effects of magnesium physiological supplementation on hyperactivity in children with attention deficit hyperactivity disorder (ADHD). Positive responses to magnesium oral loading." *Magnes Res.* 10(2):149–56, 1997.

Sterman MB & Friar L. "Suppression of Seizures in an Epileptic Following Sensorimotor EEG Feedback Training." *Electro-encephalography and Clinical Neurophysiology.* 33: 89-95, 1972.

Stevens, L, et al. "Essential fatty acids in boys with attention-deficit hyperactivity disorder." *Am J Clin Nutr.* 62: 761–8. 1995.

Stewart-Pinkham, SM. "Attention deficit disorder: a toxic response to ambient cadmium air pollution. *Int J Biosoc Med Res.* 11(2): 134–43, 1989.

"Study links sugar, child anxiety." *Chicago Tribune.* May 10, 1990.

Surwit RS. "Biofeedback: A Possible Treatment for Raynaud's Disease." In L. Birk (Ed.), Biofeedback: Behavioral Medicine. New York: Grune and Stratton. 1973.

Swain, A. et al. "Salicylates, oligoantigenic diets, and behavior." Letter to the editor. *Lancet*, pp. 41–42, July 6, 1985.

Swanson, J.M. and M. Kinsbourne. "Artificial food colors impair the learning of hyperactive children. Report to the Nutrition Foundation, 482 Fifth Avenue, New York, NY, 1979.

"Sweet Talk." *Scientific American.* Vol 257, p. 16, July 1987.

TePas, Theodore E. "Hyperactivity Revisited." *Noha News.* Vol. XIII, No. 1. Winter 1988.

Tiwari, BD et al. "Learning disabilities and poor motivation to achieve due to prolonged iron deficiency." *Am J Clin Nutr.* 63:782–6, 1996.

Tu, J-B et al. "Iron deficiency in two adolescents with Conduct, dysthymic, and movement disorders." *Can J Psychiatry.* 39:371–7, 1994.

Tuthill, RW. "Hair lead levels relation to children's classroom attention-deficit behavior. *Arch Environ Health.* 51(3):214–20, 1996.

Ullman, J. and R. *Ritalin-Free Kids: Safe and Effective Homeopathic Medicine for ADD and Other Behavioral and Learning Problems.* Prima Publishing, 1996.

Walker S III. "Drugging the American child: We're too cavalier about hyperactivity." *J. Learning Disabil.* 8: 354, 1975.

Wallis, Claudia. "Life in Overdose." *Time.* 1994, pp. 42–50, July 18.

Walter, T. "Impact of iron deficiency on cognition in infancy and childhood." *Eur J Clin Nutr.* 47:307–16, 1993.

Webb, F.F., Oski, F.A. "Iron deficiency anemia and scholastic achievement in young adolescents." *J Pediatr.* 82:827–830, 1973.

Weiss, Bernard. "Food additives as a source of behavioral disturbances in children." *Neurotoxicology.* Vol. 7, Summer pp. 197–208, 1986.

Weiss T & Engel BT. "Operant Conditioning of Heart Rate in Patients with Premature Ventricular Contractions." *Psychosomatic Medicine.* 33:310–321, 1971.

Wender, E. "Review of research on the relationship of nutritive sweeteners and behavior." In: *Diet and Behavior.* Washington, D.C.: National Center for Nutrition and Dietetics, 65–80, 1991.

Werbach, Melvyn R. *Textbook on Nutritional Medicine.* Tarzana, CA: Third Line Press, Inc., pp. 153–166, 501–8, 1999.

Whitaker, Julian. "A 'Pick-Me-Up' For Your Brain." *Health & Healing: Tomorrow's Medicine Today.* April 1992, Vol. 2, No. 4.

White, JW. And M. Wolraich. "Effect of sugar on behavior and mental performance." *Am J Clin Nutr.* 62(suppl): 242S–9S, 1995.

Wikholm, Gary. "Essential Fatty Acids: A Review of Clinical Applications." *Natural Medicine.* June 2000.

Winter, Ruth. *A Consumer's Dictionary of Food Additives.* New York: Crown, 1984.

Wolraich, M.L. et al. "Effects of diets high in sucrose or aspartame on the behavior and cognitive performance of children." *The New England Journal of Medicine.* Vol. 330, No. 5, pp. 301–307.

Wolraich, M. et al. "Effects of sucrose ingestion on the behavior of hyperactive boys." *J. Pediatrics.* 106(4):675–82, 1985.

Wolraich, ML et al. "The effect of sugar on behavior or cognition in children." *JAMA.* 274:1617–21, 1995.

Wood, David et al. "The Prevalence of Attention Deficit Disorder, Residual Type, or Minimal Brain Dysfunction, In a Population of Male Alcoholic Patients." *Am. J. Psychiatry.* 140(1):95–98, 1983.

Woodbury, MM, Woodbury, MA. "Neuropsychiatric development: two case reports about the use of dietary fish oils and/or chronic dietary supplements in children." *J Am Coll Nutr.* 12(3):239–45, 1993.

Wurtman, RJ. "Neurochemical changes following high-dose aspartame with dietary carbohydrates." *N. Engl J Med.* 309:429–30, 1983.

Yokogoski, Hidehoke et al. "Effects of Aspartame and Glucose Administration on Brain Plasma Levels of Large Neutral Amino Acids and brain 5-Hydroxindoles." *American Journal of Clinical Nutrition.* v. 40, pp. 1–7, July '84.

Zametkin, A.J., and J.L. Rappaport. "Neurobiology of Attention Deficit Disorder with Hyperactivity: Where Have We Come in 50 Years?" *J. Acad. Child and Adol. Psychiat.* 26:676–86, 1987.

Zimmerman, Marcia. "Facing Attention Deficit Disorders." *Nutrition Science News.* October 1998, Vol. 3., No. 1

CHAPTER 5

Alecson DG. *Alternative Treatments for Children Within the Autistic Spectrum.* Los Angeles: Keats Publishing. 1999.

American Psychiatric Association. *Diagnostic and Statistical Manual of Mental Disorders.* 4th ed. Washington, DC: American Psychiatric Association. 1994.

Ashraf H. "U.S. expert group rejects link between MMR and autism." *Lancet.* 357(9265):1341, Apr 28, 2001.

Autism Research Institute, 4182 Adams Street, San Diego, CA 92116. *www.autism.com*

Autism Spectrum Disorders. *http://www.geocities.com/Heartland/Fields/6979/autigen2.html.*

Baker SM, Pangborn J. *Biomedical Assessment Options: The Defeat Autism Now! (DAN!) Manual.* Autism Research Institute. 1999.

Barthelemy C, et. al. "Behavioral and biological effects of oral magnesium, vitamin B_6, and combined magnesium-B_6 administration in autistic children." *Magnesium Bulletin.* 3:150–153, 1981.

Beaupre B. "Autism Cases Skyrocket." *Chicago Sun-Times.* December 26, 2000.

Bell JG, Sargent JR, et. al. "Red blood cell fatty acid compositions in a patient with autistic spectrum disorder." a characteristic abnormality in neurodevelopmental disorders?" *ProstaglandinsLeukot Essent Fatty Acids.* 63(1/2):21–25, 2000.

Bradstreet J, El-Dahr J, et al. "Position Paper on Diagnosis and Treatment of Heavy Metal Toxicity in Autism Spectrum Disorders (ASD)." *Defeat Autism Now.* (DAN!) Subcommittee on Mercury and Autism. Draft version 1.4. Nov 2000.

Burton, Dan, Chairman-Government Reform Committee, U.S. House of Representatives. "Autism Present Challenges, Future Needs – Why the Increased Rates?" *www.house.gov/reform/hearing.../opening_statement.* April 6, 2000.

Center for Disease Control, Division of Birth Defects, Child Development and Disability Health. *http://www.cdc.gov/nceh/cddh/dd/ddautism.htm*

Chugani DC, et. al. "Developmental changes in brain serotonin synthesis capacity in autistic and non-autistic children." *Ann Neurol.* 45(3)287–95, Mar 1999.

El-Fawal HA, Gong Z, et. al. "Exposure to methyl mercury results in serum autoantibodies to neurotypic and gliotypic proteins." *Neurotoxicology.* 17(1):267–76, Spring 1996.

Feingold Association of the United States (FAUS). P.O. Box 6550, Alexandria, VA 22306. Phone: 800-321-FAUS. *www.feingold.org.*

Folstein S and Rutter M. "Infantile autism: a genetic study of 21 twin pairs." *Journal of Child Psychiatry.* 18:296–321, 1977.

Gilbert C et.al. "Folic acid as an adjunct in the treatment of children with the autism fragile-X syndrome (AFRAX)." *Med Child Neurol.* 28(5):634–7, Oct 1986.

Hoffman RL. "The Holistic MD: Autism." *Conscious Choice.* July/August 1996.

Hoshino Y et. al. "Blood serotonin and free tryptophan concentration in autistic children." *Neuropsychobiology.* 11:22–7, 1984.

Ingram JL et. al. "Discovery of allelic variants of HOXA1 and HOXB1: Genetic susceptibility to spectrum disorders." *Teratology.* 62(6):393–405, Dec 2000.

Knivsberg et. al. *Brain Dysfunct.* 3:315–327, 1990.

Lelord G, et. al. "Clinical and biological effects of vitamin B_6 + magnesium in autistic subjects." *In Leklem.*

J and Reynolds R, eds. *Vitamin B_6 Responsive Disorders in Humans.* New York: Alan R. Liss, Inc., 1988.

Lelord G, et. al. "Electrophysiological and biochemical studies in autistic children treated with vitamin B_6." In Lehmann D and Callaway E, eds. *Human Evoked Potentials: Applications and Problems.* New York: Plenum Press, 1979.

Lemer PS. "Autism: What Families Can Do." *Mothering.* 44–49, May/Jun 2000.

Lewis L. *Special Diets for Special Kids: Implementing a Diet to Improve the Lives of Children with Autism and Related Disorders.* Future Horizons. 1988.

Lowe TL et. al. "Folic acid and B_{12} in autism and neuropsychiatric disturbances of childhood." *J Am Acad Child Psychiatry.* 20(1);104–11, Winter 1981.

Maher TJ. "Neurotoxicology of Food Additives." *Neurotoxicology.* vol. 7:183–196, Summer 1986.

Malter R. "Implications of bio-nutritional approach to the diagnosis, treatment, and cost of learning disabilities." Paper presented at the Association for Children with Learning Disabilities International Conference, Washington D.C., 1983.

Marlow M, et. al. "Decreased magnesium in the hair of autistic children." *J Orthomol Psychiatry.* 13(2):177–22, 1984.

Martineau J, et. al. "Comparative effects of oral B_6, B_6-Mg, and Mg administration on evoked potentials conditioning in autistic children." In Rothenberger A, ed. *Proceedings: Symposium on Event – Related Potentials in Children.* Essen FRG 11–13 June 1982. Amsterdam: Elsevier Biomedical Press, pp. 411–416, 1982.

Martineau J, et. al. "Vitamin B_6, magnesium and combined B_6-Mg: therapeutic effects in childhood autism." *Biological Psychiatry.* 20:467-468, 1985.

Martineau J, Barthelemy C, Lelord G. "Long-term effects of combined B_6-magnesium administration in an autistic child." *Biological Psychiatry.* 21:511–518, 1986.

Martineau J, et. al. "Brief report: an open middle-term study of combined vitamin B_6 and magnesium on children with autistic behavior." *Developmental Medicine and Child Neurology.* 21:728–736, 1989.

Marshall H. "New Study fails to find link between MMR and autism." *Trends Immunol.* 22(4):185, Apr 2001.

Marwick C. "U.S. report finks no link between MMR and autism." BMJ. 5:322(7294)1083, May 2001.

Merck Research Laboratories. *The Merck Manual.* 16th ed. Rahway, NJ: Merck and Co., Inc. 1995.

Messina V. "Is NutraSweet Safe?" *Pure Facts Newsletter of the Feingold Associations of the United States.* 14(3), Apr 1990.

National Institute of Child Health and Human Development. "Vaccines and Autism: A Resource Kit." *http://www.nichd.nih.gov/publications/pubs/ autism2.htm*

National Network for Immunization Information. *http://www.immunization-info.org*

National Vaccine Information Center (NVIC) 512 W. Maple Avenue 3206, Vienna, VA 22180. Phone: 800-909-SHOT. *www.909HOT.com.*

Needleman HL. "Behavioral Toxicology." *Environ. Health Perspect. Suppl.* 6:77–9, 1995.

Options Institute: Son-Rise Program. 2080 S. Undermountain Road, Sheffield, MA 01257. Phone: 413-229-2100. *www.option.org.* or e-mail at *sonrise@option.org.*

Pfeiffer C. *Mental and Elemental Nutrients: A Guide to Nutrition and Health Care.* New Canaan: Keats, 1975.

Potenza MN, McDougle CJ. "The role of serotonin in autism-spectrum disorders." *CNS Spectrums.* 2(5):25–42, 1997.

Prohaska, Betsy. *Cooking Healthy Gluten- and Casein-Free Food for Children.* Lombard, Illinois: New Page Products. 2001. Phone: (847)-854-6601. *prohaska@mc.net*

Quigley EMM, Hurley D. "Autism and the gastrointestinal tract." [editorial]. *Am J Gastroenterol.* 95(9):2154–2156, 2000.

Reichelt et. al. *Brain Dysfunct.* 4:308–319, 1991.

Richardson AJ, Ross MA. "Fatty acid metabolism in neurodevelopmental disorders: A new perspective on associations between attention-deficit/hyperactivity disorders, dyslexia, dyspraxia and the autism spectrum." *Prostaglandins Leukot Essent Fatty Acids.* 63(1/2):1–9, 2000.

Rimland B. "Promising Approaches: What the Experts are Finding." *Mothering.* pp. 50–54, May/Jun 2000.

Rimland B. "Form Letter Regarding High Dosage Vitamin B_6 and Magnesium Therapy for Autism and Related Disorders." *Autism Research Institute.* Apr 1996.

Rimland B. "High dosage of certain vitamins in the treatment of children with severe mental disorders." In Hawkins D and Pauling L, eds. *Orthomolecular.* New York: W.H. Freeman, pp. 513–515, 1973.

Rimland B, Callaway E, Dreyfus P. "The effects of high doses of vitamin B_6 on autistic children: A double-blind cross-over study." *American Journal of Psychiatry.* 135:472–475, 1978.

Rimland B. "Megavitamin B_6 and magnesium in the treatment of autistic children and adolescents." In Schopler E and Mesibov GB, eds. *Neurobiological Issues in Autism.* New York: Plenum Press, pp. 389–405, 1987.

Rimland B and Larson G. "Hair mineral analysis and behavior: analysis of 51 studies." *Journal of Learning Disabilities.* 16:279-285, May 1983.

Rimland B. *Infantile Autism.* Englewood Cliffs, New Jersey: Prentice Hall. 1964.

Roberts R. "MMR vaccination and autism. There is no causal link between MMR vaccine and autism." *BMJ.* 13:316(7147):1824. Jun 1998.

Rossi P, Visconti P, Bergossi A, Balcatra V. "Effects of vitamin B_6 and magnesium therapy in autism." Conference on the Neurobiology of Infantile Autism, Tokyo, Japan, Nov 10-11, 1990.

Rutter M and Bartak L. "Causes of infantile autism: Some considerations from recent research." *Journal of Autism and Childhood Schizophrenia.* 1:20–32, 1971.

Sassen AN et. al. "Neuroimminotoxicology: Humoral Assessment of Neurotoxicity and Autoimmune Mechanisms." *Environ. Health Perspect.* Vol. 107. Suppl. Oct. 5, 1999.

Schutt CE. "Secretin and Autism: A Clue But Not a Cure." *NAARRATIVE: Newsletter of the National Alliance for Autism Research.* No. 4, Winter 1998.

Schwartz MW, Curry TA, Sargent AJ, et. al. *Pediatric Primary Care.* 3rd ed. St. Louis, Missouri: Mosby-Year Book, Inc. 1997.

Singh VK et. al. "Antibodies to myelin basic protein in children with autistic behavior." *Brain Behav Immun.* 7(1):97:103, Mar 1993.

Smeeth L et. al. "Measles, mumps and rubella (MMR) vaccine and autism. Ecological studies answer main question." *BMJ.* 323(7305):163, Jul 21, 2001.

Ullman J and Ullman R. *Ritalin-Free Kids: Safe and Effective Homeopathic Medicine for ADD and Other Behavioral and Learning Problems.* Rocklin, California: Prima Publishing. 1996.

Upledger Institute, Inc. *Cranial Sacral Therapy.*, 11211 Prosperity Farms Road, Suite D-325, Palm Beach, FL 33410. Phone: 516-622-4334. *upledger@upledger.com.*

Vastag B. "Congressional autism hearings continue: No evidence MMR vaccine causes disorder." *JAMA.* 285(20):2567–9, May 23-30, 2001.

Wakefield AJ, Anthony A, et. al. "Enterocolitis in Children with Developmental Disorders." *Am J Gastroenterol.* 95(9):2285–2295, 2000.

Werbach MR. *Textbook of Nutritional Medicine.* Tarzana, California: Third Line Press, Inc. 1999.

CHAPTER 6

"Adverse Drug Reactions." *The Sunday Herald* (London), December 10 & 17, 2000.

Alm JS et al. "Atopy in children of families with an anthroposophic lifestyle." *Lancet.* 353:1485-1488, 1999.

Asa PB., Cao Y., Garry R. Antibodies to squalene in Gulf War Syndrome. *Experimental and Molecular Pathology.* 68(1):55–64, February 2000.

Barclay, et al. "Research from the south, vitamin A supplements and mortality related to measles: a randomized clinical trial." *British Medical Journal.* Jan. 31, 1987.

Beeson, P., et al. "Hepatitis following injection of mumps convalescent plasma." *Lancet.* 814–816, June 24, 1944.

Benjamin, C.M., et al. "Joint and limb symptoms in children after immunization with measles, mumps, and rubella vaccine." *British Medical Journal.* 1075–1078, April 25, 1992

Christie, CDC, et al. "The 1993 epidemic of pertussis in Cincinnati- resurgence of disease in a highly immunized population of children." *New England Journal of Medicine.* Vol. 331, No. 1, July 7, 1994.

Coulter H. *Divided Legacy: The conflict between homeopathy and the American Medical Association.* Berkely, California: North Atlantic Books. 1973.

Coulter, Harris L. and Fisher, Barbara. *DPT: A Shot in the Dark.* New York: Warner Books, 1985.

Department of Defense news briefing. October 4, 2000. Available from M2 Communications (*www.m2.com*).

Digestive Disorder Science, 45(4):723-9, April 2000.

DPT (Dissatisfied Parents Together). For information: (703) 938-DPT3.

Dunbar, Bonnie, Ph.D. For information: (web pages.*netlink.co.nzias dunbar.htm*)

Eisenstein, Mayer, M.D., J.D., M.P.H. *Safer Medicine.* Chicago: CMI Press, 2000.

Eriksson P. "Developmental neurotoxicity of environmental agents in the neonate." *Neurotoxicology.* 18(3):719–726, 1997.

Evenson AJ, Martin T. "Medical examiner links death to anthrax vaccine." *Lansing State Journal.* September 28, 2000.

Fitzgerald WF, Clarks TW. "Mercury and monomethylmercury: Present and future concerns." *Environmental Health Perspective.* 96:159–166. 1991.

Garenne, Michel, et al. "Child mortality after high-titre measles vaccines: prospective study in Snegal." *Lancet.* Vol.338:903–907, Oct. 12, 1991.

Gaucher C, Jeulin D, Peycru P. "Homeopathic treatment of cholera in Peru: an initial clinical study." *Brit Homeop J.* 81:18–21, 1992.

Gilbert SG, Grant-Webster KS. *Neurobehavioral Effects of Developmental Methylmercury Exposure. Environmental Health Perspective.* 103 (Suppl 6): 135–142, 1995.

"Government now admits traces of chemical in anthrax vaccines." *Alternative Medicine Newsletter.* October 6, 2000.

Grandjean P, Weihe P, White R, et al. "{Cognitive Deficit in 7-Year Old children with prenatal exposure to methylmercury." *Neurotoxicol Teratol.* 1997:19(6):417–428.

Herroelen, L. et al. "Central Nervous System demelination after immunization with recombinent Hepatitis B vaccine." *Lancet.* Volume 338, 1174–1175, 1991.

Honeyman MC, et al. "Association between rotavirus infection and pancreatic islet autoimmunity in children at risk of developing type I diabetes." *Diabetes.* August 49(8):1319–24, 2000.

Honeyman MC, Brusic V, Stone N, Harrison LC. "Neural network-based prediction of candidate T-cell epitopes." *Nature Biotechnology.* October 16(10):966, 1998.

Illinois Vaccine Awareness Coalition (IVAC). P.O. Box 946, Oak Park, IL 60303.

Incao P. "Supporting children's health." *Alternative Medicine Digest.* Issue 19, 54–59, 1997.

Journal of Adverse Drug Reactions. England; November 2000 (Volume 19, Issue 4).

Kemp T et al. "Is infant immunization a risk factor for childhood asthma or allergy?" *Epidemiology.* 8(6): 678–680, 1997.

Keusch, Gerald T. "Vitamin A supplements- too good to not be true." *The New England Journalof Medicine.* 985-987, October 4, 1990.

Landrigan, P., White, J. "Neurologic disorders following live measles virus vaccination." *Journal of the American Medical Association.* Volume 223, No. 13:1459–62, 1973.

Mair, I., Leverland, H. "Sudden deafness and vaccination." *Journal of Laryngology and Otology.* Volume 91:323–29, 1977.

Mendelsohn, Robert S. *Confessions of a Medical Heretic.* Chicago: Contemporary Books, 1979.

Mendelsohn, Robert S., M.D. *How to Raise a Healthy Child in Spite of Your Doctor.* Chicago: Contemporary Books, Inc. 1984.

Miller, H., et al. "Multiple sclerosis and vaccination." *British Medical Journal.* 210-13, 1967.

National Coalition for Adult Immunization. (301) 656-0003. *www.nfid.org/ncal.*

National Research Council. *Pesticides in the Diets of Infants and Children.* Washington DC: National Academy Press, 1993.

National Vaccine Information Center. phone #: (800) 999-7468. or website: *www.909shot.com*

Neustaedter, Randall, OMD. *The Vaccine Guide: Making An Informed Choice.* Berkeley: North Atlantic Books, 1996.

NOHA Newsletter. *Vaccines.* Thomas L. Stone, M.D., page 5.

Odent MR. "Pertussis vaccination and asthma: Is there a link?" *JAMA,* 271:229-231, 1994.

Ogra. P., Herd, K. "Arthritis associated with induced rubella infection." *Journal of Immunology.* Volume 107, 810–13, 1971.

Sheneen SO et al. "Measles and atopy in Guinea-Bissau." *Lancet.* 1996; 347:1792–1796.

Weiss B, Reuhl K. *Delayed Neurotoxicity.* Louis W. Chang, ed. Marcel Dekker, New York, publisher, 1994.

CHAPTER 7

Arnaud CD, et al. "The Role of Calcium in Osteoporosis." *Annu Rev Nutr.* 397-413, 1990.

Bachrach LK. "Acquisition of optimal bone mass in childhood and adolescence." *Trends Endocrinol Metab.* 12:22–28, 2001.

Bryant RJ, Cadogan J, Weaver CM. "The new dietary reference intakes for calcium: Implications for osteoporosis." *J Am Coll Nutr.* 18(5 Suppl):406S–412S, Oct 1999.

Carrie Fassler AL., Bonjour JP. "Osteoporosis as a pediatric problem." *Pediatr Clin North Am.* 42:811–824, 1995.

Cromer B, Hasel Z. "Adolescents: at risk for osteoporosis?" *Clin Pediatr.* 39:565–574, 2000.

Dempster DW, Lindsay R. "Pathogenesis of osteoporosis." *Lancet.* 341:797–805, 1993.

Dhuper S, Warren MP, Brooks-Gunn J, Fox R. "Effects of hormonal status on bone density in adolescent girls." *J Clin Endocrinol Metab.* 71:1083–1088, 1990.

Eberle J, Schmidmayer S, Erben RG, et. al. "Skeletal effects of zinc deficiency on growing rats." *J Trace Elem Med Biol.* 13:21–26, 1999.

El-Hajj Fuleihan G, Nabulsi M, Choucair M. "Hypovitaminosis D in healthy schoolchildren." *Pediatrics.* 107(4), 2001.

Fleming, KH and Heimbach JT. "Consumption of Calcium in the U.S.: Food Sources and Intake Levels." *Amer Inst Nutr.* 1426S–1430S, 1994.

Food and Nutrition Board, Institute of Medicine. *Dietary Reference Intakes (DRIs) for Calcium, Phosphorus, Magnesium, Vitamin D, and Fluoride.* Washington DC: National Academy Press. 1997.

Frost HM. "Changing views about 'Osteoporosis' (a 1998 overview)." *Osteoporos Int.* 10(5):345–352, 1999.

Frost HM. "The 'muscle-bone unit' in children and adolescents: A 2000 overview." *J Pediatr Endocrinol Metab.* 13(6):571–590, Jun 2000.

Fuller KE, Casparian JM. "Vitamin D: Balancing cutaneous and systemic considerations." *South Med J.* 94(1):58–64, Jan 2001.

Hampl JS and Betts NM. "Cigarette use during adolescence: effects on nutritional status." *Nutr Rev.* 57(7):215–221, Jul 2000.

Hansen MA, Overgaard K, Riis BJ, Christensen C. "Role of peak bone mass and bone loss in postmenopausal osteoporosis: 12 year study." *Br Med J.* 303:961–964, 1991.

Haas EM. *Staying Healthy with the Seasons.* Berkley, California: Celestial Arts. 1981.

Heaney RP. "Thinking straight about calcium." *N Engl J Med.* 328:503–505, 1993.

Horwath C, Parnell WR, Wilson NC, Russell DG. "Attaining optimal bone status: lessons from the 1997 National Nutrition Survey." *N Z Med J.* 114(1128):138–141, Mar 23, 2001.

Hustmyer FG, Peacock M, Hui S, et. al. "Bone mineral density in relation to polymorphism at the vitamin D receptor gene locus." *J Clin Invest.* 94:2130–2134, 1994.

Igarashi A., Yamaguchi M. "Increase in bone protein components with healing rat fractures: Enhancement by zinc treatment." *Int J Mol Med.* 4:615–620, 1999.

Kasper MJ, Peterson MG, Allegrante JP, et. al. "Knowledge, beliefs, and behaviors among college women concerning the prevention of osteoporosis." *Arch Fam Med.* 3(8):696–702, Aug 1994.

Lark S. "Bountiful Bone Part I" The Lark Letter-Empowering Women, *Restoring Health.* vol. 8 no. 5.

Linder MC. "Nutrition and Metabolism of the Major Minerals." *Nutritional Biochemistry and Metabolism with Clinical Applications.* 2nd ed. East Norwalk, Connecticut: Appleton & Livingstone. 1999.

Lindsay R. "Prevention and treatment of osteoporosis." *Lancet.* 341:801–805, March 27, 1993.

Lloyd T, Andon MB, Rollings N, et. al. "Calcium supplementation and bone mineral density in adolescent girls." *JAMA.* 270:841–844, 1993.

Marz, RB. *Medical Nutrition from Marz.* 2nd ed., Portland, Oregon: Omni-Press. 1997.

Massey, LK. "Acute effects of dietary caffeine and sucrose on urinary mineral excretion in healthy adolescents." *Nutr Res.* 8(9), 1988.

Matsuoka LY, Wortsman J, Hollis BW. "Suntanning and cutaneous synthesis of vitamin D_3." *J Lab Clin Med.* 116:87–90, 1990.

Meunier PJ. "Is steroid-induced osteoporosis preventable?" *N Engl J Med.* 328:1781–1782, Jun 17, 1993. Editorials.

Moon J, Bandy B, Davison AJ. "Hypothesis: Etiology of atherosclerosis and osteoporosis. Are imbalances in the calciferol endocrine system implicated?" *J Am Coll Nutr.* 11:567–83, 1992.

Murray MT. "Osteoporosis Prevention and Treatment – Beyond Calcium." *Natural Medicine Journal.* 2(5)5–12, 1999.

Murray, MT. "Bone Health." Ask the Doctor. Vital Communications, Inc. 1999.

Pizzorno JE, Murray MT. *Textbook of Natural Medicine.* 2nd ed., London: Churchill Lange. pp.191–214, 1991.

Rozen GS, Rennert G, Rennert HS, et. al. "Calcium intake and bone mass development among Israeli adolescent girls." *Journal of the American College of Nutrition.* 20(3):219–224, Jun 2001.

Sabatier JP, Guaydier-Souquieres G, Laroche D, et. al. "Bone mineral acquisition during adolescence and early childhood: a study in 574 healthy females 10–24-years-old." *Osteoporos Int.* 6:141–148, 1996.

Saltman P, Strause LG. "The role of trace minerals in osteoporosis." *J Amer Coll Nutr.* 12(4):384–389, 1993.

Sasaki M., Harata S., Kumasawa Y., et. al. "Bone mineral density and osteo sono assessment index in adolescents." *J Orthop Sci.* 5:185–191, 2000.

Sentipal JM, Wardlaw GM, Mahan J, et. al. "Influence of calcium intake and growth indexes on vertebral bone mineral density in young females." *Am J Clin Nutr.* 54:425–428, 1991.

Shils ME, Olson JA, Shike M, Ross AC. eds. *Modern Nutrition in Health and Disease.* 9th ed. New York: Lippincott Williams & Wilkins. 1999.

Sojka JE. "Magnesium supplementation and osteoporosis." *Nutr Rev.* 53(3):71–4, 1995.

Turner JG, Gilchrist NL, Ayling EM, et. al. "Factors affecting bone mineral density in high school girls." *NZ Med J.* 105:95–97, 1992.

Vieth R. "Vitamin D supplementation, 25-hydroxyvitamin D concentrations, and safety." *Am J Clin Nutr.* 69:842–856, 1999.

Weaver CM. "Age related calcium requirements due to changes in absorption and utilization." *J Nutr.* 124:1418S–1425S, 1994.

Weaver CM, Peacock M, Johnston CC. "Adolescent nutrition in the prevention of postmenopausal osteoporosis." *J Clin Endocrinol Metab.* 84:1839–1843, 1999.

CHAPTER 8

American Academy of Pediatrics. "Rise in Childhood Obesity Linked to Increase in Type-2 Diabetes." Press release. February 23, 2000.

American Anorexia Bulimia Association, 165 West 46th Street, Suite 1108, New York, NY 10036. Phone: 212-575-6200. *www.aabainc.org*

American Diabetes Association. "Type 2 diabetes in children and adolescents." *Pediatrics.* 105(3):671-680, Mar 2000.

American Psychiatric Association. Diagnostic and Statistical Manual of Mental Disorders. 4th ed. Washington, DC: American Psychiatric Association. 1994.

Andersen AE, DiDomenico L. "Diet vs. shape content of popular male and female magazines: A dose response relationship to the incidence of eating disorders?" *International Journal of Eating Disorders.* 11(3):283–287, 1992.

Andersen AE, Holman JE. "Males with eating disorders: Challenges for treatment and research." *Psychopharmacology Bulletin.* 33(3):391-397, 1977.

Begley S. "What families should do: Helping children lose weight means walking an emotional tightrope. How, and when, to step in." *Newsweek.* pp. 44–47, July 3, 2000.

Birch LL, Davison KK. "Family environmental factors influencing the developing behavioral controls of food intake and childhood overweight." *Pediatr Clin North Am.* 48(4):893–907, Aug 2001.

Carlat DJ, Carmago CA. "Review of bulimia nervosa in males." *American Journal of Psychiatry.* 148:831–843, 1991.

Center for Science in the Public Interest. "Diet & Health: Ten Megatrends." *Nutrition Action Healthletter.* Jan/Feb 2001.

Condor B. "The fat fact: Increasing numbers of kids are weighed down by obesity." *Chicago Tribune.* October 3, 1999.

Collins ME. "Body figure perceptions and preferences among pre-adolescent children." *International Journal of Eating Disorders.* 10(2):199–208, 1991.

Cowley G. "Generation XXL: Childhood obesity now threatens one in three kids with long-term health, problems, and the crisis is growing." *Newsweek.* July 3, 2000. pp. 40–44.

Cowley G, Begley S. "Fat for life? Six million kids are seriously overweight. What families can do." *Newsweek.* July 3, 2000. pp. 40–47.

Fairburn CG, Beglin SJ. "Studies of the epidemiology of bulimia nervosa." *American Journal of Psychiatry.* 147(4):401–408, 1990.

Gustafson-Larson A, Terry RD. "Weight-related behaviors and concerns of fourth-grade children." *Journal of the American Dietetic Association.* 92:818–822, 1992.

Hellmich N. "Kids gobbling empty calories. All this nibbling round the clock is adding to concerns about obesity." *USA Today.* April 30, 2001.

Hill AJ, Draper E, Stack,J. "A weight on children's minds: Body shape dissatisfactions at 9-years old." *International Journal of Obesity and Related Metabolic Disorders.* 18(6):383–389, 1994.

Killen JD, Taylor CB, Telch MJ, et. al. "Self-induced vomiting and laxative and diuretic use among teenagers: Precursors of the binge-purge syndrome?" *JAMA.* 255:1447–1449, 1986.

Kohn M, Golden NH. "Eating disorders in children and adolescents: Epidemiology, diagnosis and treatment." *Paediatr Drugs.* 3(2):91–99, 2001.

MacBrayer EK, Smith GT, McCarthy DM, et. al. "The role of family of origin food-related experiences in bulimic symptomatology." *Int J Eat Disord.* 30(2):149–160, Sep 2001.

Mintz LB, Betz NE. "Prevalence and correlates of eating disordered behaviors among undergraduate women." *Journal of Counseling Psychology.* 35(4):463–471, 1988.

Mellin LM, Irwin CE, Scully S. "Prevalence of disorder eating in girls: A survey of middle-class children." *Journal of the American Dietetic Association.* 92:851–853, 1992.

Mokdad AH, Serdula MK, Dietz WH, et. al. "The spread of the obesity epidemic in the United States, 1991–1998." *JAMA.* 282(16):1519–1522, Oct 27, 1999.

National Association of Anorexia Nervosa and Associated Disorders (ANAD), PO Box 7, Highland Park, IL 60035 Hotline: 847-831-3438 *www.anad.org*

National Center for Health Statistics, Division of Data Services, Hyattsville, MD 20782-2003. Phone (301) 458-4636 *www.cdc.gov/nchs*

National Institute of Mental Health. *Eating Disorders: Facts About Eating Disorders and the Search for Solutions.* NIH Publication No. 01-4901, Rockville, Maryland. 2001.

Nemeroff CJ, Stein RI, Diehl NS, Smilack KM. "From the Cleavers to the Clintons: Role choices and body orientation as reflected in magazine article content." *International Journal of Eating Disorders.* 16(2):167–176, 1994.

Reno EG. "Eating disorders and food addictions." *The Nutrition & Dietary Consultant.* Feb 1992.

Robin AL. "A controlled comparison of family versus individual therapy for adolescents with anorexia nervosa." *J Amer Acad Child Adolesc Psychiatry.* 38(12):1482–1489, 1999.

Rosen MD. "Adult problems reach preteens. Victims of eating disorders are getting younger and younger." *Chicago Tribune.* September 17, 2000.

St. Joseph Medical Center, 7601 Osler Drive, Towson, Maryland 21204-7582 Phone 410-337-1000. *www.sjmcmd.org*

Schwartz MW, Curry TA, Sargent AJ, et. al. *Pediatric Primary Care: A Problem-Oriented Approach.* 3rd ed. St. Louis, Missouri: Mosby-Yearbook, Inc. 1997.

Serdula MK, Collins E, Williamson DF, et. al. "Weight control practices of US adolescents and adults." *Annals of Internal Medicine.* 119:667–671, 1993.

Shepard K. *From the First Bite: A Complete Guide to Recovering from Food Addiction.* Deerfield Beach, Florida: Health Communications, Inc. 2000.

Strober M, Freeman R, Lampert C, et. al. "Males with anorexia nervosa: a controlled study of eating disorders in first-degree relatives." *Int J Eat Disord.* 29(3):263–269, Apr 2001.

Sullivan PF. "Mortality in Anorexia Nervosa." *American Journal of Psychiatry.* 152(7):1073–1074, 1995.

Tierney LM, McPhee SJ, Papadakis MA. *Current Medical Diagnosis & Treatment.* New York: Lange Medical Books/McGraw-Hill. 2000.

Woodside DB, Garfinkel PE, Lin E, et. al. "Comparisons of men with full or partial eating disorders, men without eating disorders, and women with eating disorders in the community." *Am J Psychiatry.* 158(4):570–574, Apr 2001.

CHAPTER 9

Almeida JC, Grimsley EW. "Coma from the Health Food Store: Interaction between Kava and Alprazolam." *Ann Int Med.* 125(11): 940, 1996.

Altonn H. "Prozac's role in Maui deaths going to court: A family that suffered a murder-suicide sues the maker of the drug." *Honolulu Star-Bulletin.* Jan 9, 1998.

American Psychiatric Association. *Diagnostic and Statistical Manual of Mental Disorders.* 4th ed. (DSM-IV). Washington DC: American Psychiatric Press. 1994.

Bellafante G. "How Could He Have Done It? Michael Hutchence's Baffling Death Is The Latest Chapter In A Rock-'N'-Roll Romance Lived In Excess." *Time Magazine.* Dec 8, 1997.

Birmaher B, Ryan ND, Williamson DE, et.al. "Childhood and adolescent depression: a review of the past 10 years. Part 1." *Journal of the American Academy of Child and Adolescent Psychiatry.* 35(11):1427–39, 1996.

Boergers J, Spirito A, Donaldson D. "Reasons for adolescent suicide attempts: Associations with psychological functioning." *Journal of the American Academy of Child and Adolescent Psychiatry.* 37:1287–93, 1998.

Brent DA, Holder D, Kolko D. et. al. "A clinical psychotherapy trial for adolescent depression comparing cognitive, family, and supportive therapy." *Archives of General Psychiatry.* 54(9):877–85, 1997.

Brinker F. *The Toxicology of Botanical Medicines.* 2nd ed. Sandy, Oregon: Eclectic Medical Pub. 1996.

Brockmoller J, Reum T, Bauer S, et. al. "Hypericin and Pseudohypericin: Pharmokinetics and Effects on Photosensitivity in Humans." *Pharmacopsychiat.* 30:94–101, 1997.

Brooks S. ed. "Botanical Toxicology." *Protocol J Bot Med.* 1(1):147–58, 1995.

Brophy B. "Kindergartners in the Prozac nation." U.S. News Online. Nov 13, 1995. *www.usnews.com/usnews/issue/prozac*

Brown J, Cohen P, Johnson JG, et. al. "Childhood abuse and neglect: specificity of effects on adolescent and young adult depression and suicidality." *Journal of the American Academy of Child and Adolescent Psychiatry.* 38(12):1490–6, 1999.

Brown R. "Potential interactions of herbal medicines with antipsychotics, antidepressants and hypnotics." *Eur J Herb Med.* 3(2):25–8, 1997.

De Smet PAGM, et. al. (eds.) *Adverse Effects of Herb Drugs 2.* Berlin: Springer-Verlag, 1993.

Farnsworth NR, Bingel AS, Cordell GA, Crane FA, Fong HHS. "Potential Value of Plants as Sources of New Antifertility Agents I". *J Pharm Sci.* 64:535–98, 1975.

Feingold Association of the United States (FAUS). P.O. Box 6550, Alexandria, VA 22306. 800-32-FAUS. *www.feingold.org.*

Fetrow CW, Avila JR. *Professional's Handbook of Complementary & Alternative Medicines.* Springhouse, Pennsylvania: Springhouse Corporation. 1999.

Field T, Lang C. Yando R, Bendell D. "Adolescents' intimacy with parents and friends." *Adolescence.* 30:133–140, 1995.

Fleming JE, Offord DR. "Epidemiology of childhood depressive disorders: A critical review." *Journal of the American Academy of Child and Adolescent Psychiatry.* 29(4):571–80, 1990.

Gaby AR. "Why All the Violence? (Prozac and other selective serotonin-reuptake inhibitors (SSRI))." *Townsend Letter for Doctors and Patients.* May 2001.

Geller B, Reising D, Leonard HL, et. al. "Critical review of tricyclic antidepressant use in children and adolescents." *Journal of the American Academy of Child and Adolescent Psychiatry.* 38(5):513–6, 1999.

Gruenwald J, Brendler T, Jaenicke C. eds. *Physician's Desk Reference for Herbal Medicines.* 1st ed. Montvale, New Jersey: Medical Economics Company. 1998.

Harrer G, Hubner WD, Podzuweit H. "Effectiveness and tolerance multicenter double-blind study." *J Geriatr Psychiatry Neurol.* 7(suppl 1):S24–28, 1994.

Herberg KW. "The influence of kava-special extract WS 1490 on safety-relevant performance alone and in combination with ethylalcohol." *Blutalkohol.* 30:96–105, 1993.

Holzl J, Demisch L, Gollnik B. "Investigations about antidepressive and mood changing effects of *Hypericum perforatum.*" *Planta Med.* 55:643, 1989.

Hurd KP, Wooding S, Noller P. "Parent-adolescent relationships in families with depressed and self-harming adolescents." *Journal of Family Studies.* 5:47–68, 1999.

Jamieson DD, Duffield PH. "Positive interaction of ethanol and kava resin in mice." *Clin Exp. Pharmacol. Physiol.* 17:509–14, 1990.

Jamieson DD, Duffield PH, Cheng D, Duffield AM. "Comparison of the central nervous system activity of the activity of the aqueous and lipid extract of kava (Piper methysticum)." *Arch Int Pharmacodyn Ther.* 301:66–80, (C.A. 11291628f) 1989.

Jussofie A, Schmiz A, Hiemke C. "Kavapyrone enriched extract from Piper methysticum as modulator of the GABA binding site in different regions of rat brain." *Psychopharm.* 116:469–74, 1994.

Kaslow NJ, Deering CGR, Racusin G. "Depressed children and their families." *Clinical Psychology Review.* 14:39–59, 1994.

Kenworthy T, Priest D. "Littleton Shooter Was Rejected by Marines." *Washington Post.* Apr 28, 1999.

Kinzler E, Kromer J, Lehmann E. "Clinical efficacy of a kava controlled study over 4 weeks." *Arzneim Forsch.* 41:584–588, 1991.

Klein DN, Lewinsohn PM, Seeley JR, Rohde P. "A family study of major depressive disorder in a community sample of adolescents." *Archives of General Psychiatry.* 58:13–20, 2001.

Klerman GL, Weissman MM. "Increasing rates of depression." *Journal of the American Medical Association.* 261:2229–35, 1989.

Knox M, King C, Hanna GL, Logan D, Ghaziuddin N. "Progressive behavior in clinically depressed adolescents." *Journal of the American Academy of Child and Adolescent Psychiatry.* 39(5):611–618, May 2000.

Lewinsohn PM, Rohde P, Seeley JR. "Major depressive disorder in older adolescents: Prevalence, risk factors, and clinical implication." *Clinical Psychology Review.* 18(7):765–94, 1998.

Linde K, Ramirez G, Mulrow CD, et. al. "St. John's wort for depression – an overview and meta-analysis of randomized clinical trials." *Br Med J.* 313:253–8, 1996.

Lindenberg D, Pitule-Schodel H. "D,L-kavain in comparison with oxazepam in anxiety disorders. A double-blind study of clinical effectiveness." *Forschr Med.* 108:49–50, 53–54, 1990.

McGuffin M, Hobbs C, Upton R, Goldberg A. eds. *Botanical Safety Handbook.* Boca Raton: CRC Press.1997.

Monroe SM, Rohde P, Seeley JR, et. al. "Life events and depression in adolescents: relationship loss as a prospective risk factor for first onset of major depressive disorder." *Journal of Abnormal Psychology.* 108(4):606–14, 1999.

Moore TJ. *Prescription for Disaster. The Hidden Dangers in Your Medicine Cabinet.* Simon & Schuster. 1998.

Mufson L, Weissman MM, Moreau D, et. al. "Efficacy od interpersonal psychotherapy for depressed adolescents." *Archives of General Psychiatry.* 56(6):573–9, 1999.

Munte TF, Heinze HJ, Matzke M. "Effects of oxazepam and an extract of kava roots (piper methysticum) on event-related potentials in a word recognition task." *Neuropyschobiol.* 27:46–53, 1993.

National Institutes of Mental Health. *Depression in Children and Adolescents: A Fact Sheet for Physicians.* NIH Publication No. 00-4744. Available from NIMH, 6001 Executive Boulevard, Room 8184, MSC 9663, Bethesda, MD 20892-9663.

Okpanyi SN, Weischer ML. "Experimental animal studies of the psychotropic activity of a hypericum extract." *Arzneim.-Forsch.* 37:10–13, 1987.

Physician's Desk Reference. 54th ed. 2000, pp. 962-966.

Pizzorno JE, Murray MT. eds. *Textbook of Natural Medicine.* 2nd ed. London: Churchhill Livingstone 1999.

Prozac Survivors Support Group. *www.pssg.org*

Ronzio RA. *The Encyclopedia of Nutrition & Good Health.* New York: Facts On File, Inc. 1997.

Ryan ND, Puig-Antich J, Ambrosini P, et. al. "The clinical picture of major depression in children and adolescents." *Archives of General Psychiatry.* 44:854–61, 1987.

Schelosky L, Raffauf C, Jendroska K, Poewe W. "Kava and dopamine antagonism." *J Neurol Neurosurg Psychiatry,* 58(5):639–40, 1995.

Shaffer D, Craft L. "Methods of adolescent suicide prevention." *Journal of Clinical Psychiatry.* 60(Suppl 2): 70–4; discussion 75–6, 133–6, 1999.

Shaffer D, Gould MS, Fisher P, et. al. "Psychiatric diagnosis in child and adolescent suicide." *Archives of General Psychiatry.* 53(4):339–48, 1996.

Shiner RL, Marmorstein NR. "Family environments of adolescents with lifetime depression: Associations with maternal depression history." *Journal of the American Academy of Child and Adolescent Psychiatry.* 37:1152–1160, 1998.

Silver ME. "Angry adolescents who worry about becoming violent." *Adolescence.* Winter 2000.

Silverman JG. "Physical and sexual abuse of teen girls by a dating partner." *JAMA.* Aug 2001.

Singh Y. "Kava: an overview." *J Ethnopharmacol.* 37:13–45, 1992.

Swenson J. "Man convicted of driving under influence of kava." *Desert News.* Aug 5, 1996.

Thomas CL. ed. *Taber's Cyclopedic Medical Dictionary.* St. Louis, Missouri: F.A. Davis Company. 1993.

Tursi R, Wiersma A, Hughes KK. "Binge-drinking-related consequences in college students: Role of drinking beliefs and mother-teen communications." *Psychology of Addictive Behaviors.* Vol. 14, No. 4.

Twenge JM. "Today's children experience more anxiety." *Journal of Personality and Social Psychology.* 79(6):1007–1021, Dec 2000.

Valois RE, McKewon RE. "Frequency and correlates of fighting and carrying weapons among public school adolescents." *American Journal of Health Behavior.* 22:8–17, 1998.

Vorbach EU, Arnoldt KH, Hubner W-D. "Efficacy and tolerability of St. John's wort extract LI 160 versus imipramine in patients with severe depressive episodes according to ICE-10." *Pharmacopsychiat.* 30(suppl):81–85, 1997.

Weinberg WA, Harper CR, Emslie GJ, Brumback RA. "Depression and other affective illnesses as a cause of school failure and maladaptation in learning disabled children, adolescents, and young adults." *Secondary Education and Beyond: Providing Opportunity for Students with Learning Disabilities.* Learning Disabilities Association of America Press. pp. 234–264, 1995.

Weissman MM, Wolk S, Goldstein RB, et. al. "Depressed adolescents grown up." *Journal of the American Medical Association.* 281:1701–13, 1999.

Wells VE, Deykin EY, Kleman GL. "Risk factors for depression in older adolescents. *Psychiatric Development.* 3(1):83-108, 1985.

Werbach MR. *Textbook of Nutritional Medicine.* Tarzana, California: Third Line Press, Inc. 1999.

Whitaker J. "The Scourge of Prozac." *Health & Healing* Vol.9, No. 9. September, 1999.

Wichtl M. ed. *Herbal Drugs and Phytopharmaceuticals.* Boca Raton: CRC Press. 1994.

Wills TA, McNamara G, Vaccaro D, Hirky E. "Escalated substance use: A longitudinal grouping analysis from early to middle adolescence." *Journal of Abnormal Psychology.* 105(2):166–180, 1999.

CHAPTER 10

Acheson LS, Harris SE, Zyzanski, SJ. "Patient Selection and outcomes for out-of-hospital births in one family practice." *Journal of Family Practice.* 31:128–36, 1990.

Ackerman-Liebrich U, Voegli I, Guenther-Wittk, etc al. "Home versus hospital deliveries: a prospective study on matched pairs." *British Medical Journal.* 313:1313–18, 1996.

American Academy of Pediatrics. "Breastfeeding and the use of human milk." *Pediatrics.* 100:1035–9, 1997.

American College of Obstetricians and Gynecologists. *Evaluation of Cesarean Delivery.* Washington D.C.: ACOG, 2000.

Amu O, Rajendran S. Bolaji I. "Should Doctors Perform and Elective Cesarean Section on Request? Maternal Choice Alone Should Not Determine Method of Delivery." *British Medical Journal.* 317:463–465, 1998.

Belizan, D. "Routine vs. selective episiotomy: a randomized controlled trial." *Lancet.* 342:1517–18, 1993.

Caudill, Marie. "Current and Emerging Issue in Folate Nutriture." *Nutrition Today.* Vol. 35, No. 6: 206-209, 2000.

Cullen C, Field T, Escalona A, Hartshorn K. (In Review.) "Father-infant interactions are enhanced by massage therapy." *Spine.*

Davies J, Hey E, Reid W, et al. "Prospective regional study of planned homebirth." *British Medical Journal.* 313:1302–5, 1996.

Eisenstein, Mayer. *Homebirth Advantage.* Chicago: CMI Press, 2000.

Eisentstein, Mayer. Safer Medicine. Chicago: CMI Press, 2000, pp. 1–110.

Eisenberg, Arlene et al. *What to Expect When You're Expecting.* New York: Workman Publishing Co., 1991.

Ewingman, Bernard. "Effects of prenatal ultrasound screening on perinatal outcome." *New England Journal of Medicine.* September 16, 1993; Vol. 329: 821–7.

"Frequent prenatal ultrasound: time to think again." *Lancet.* Vol. 342: 878, October 1993.

Field T. *Touch Therapy.* London: Churchill Livingstone. 2000.

Field T, Henteleff T, Hernandez-Reif M, et. al. "Children with asthma have improved pulmonary functions after massage therapy." *Journal of Pediatrics.* 132:854–858, 1998.

Field T, Hernandez-Reif M, Hart S, Theakston H. "Pregnant women benefit from massage therapy." *Journal of Psychosomatic Obstetrics and Gynecology.* 19, 1999.

Field T, Hernandez-Reif M, LeGreca A, et. al. "Massage therapy lowers blood glucose levels in children with Diabetes Mellitus." *Diabetes Spectrum.* 10:237–239, 1997.

Field T, Kilmer T, Hernandez-Reif M, Burman I. "Preschool children's sleep and wake behavior improve after massage therapy." *Early Child Development & Care.* 120:39–44, 1997.

Field T, Lasko D, Mundy P, et. al. "Autistic children's attentiveness and responsivity improved after touch therapy." *Journal of Autism & Developmental Disorders.* 27:333–338, 1997.

FuKushima Y, Kawata Y, Onda T, Kitagawa M. "Consumption of cow milk and egg by lactating woman and the presence of beta-lactoglobulin and ovabumin in breast milk." *American Journal of Medicine.* 327: 380–4, 1992.

Goldman AS. "The immune system of human milk: antimicrobial, antiinflammatory and Immunomodulating properties." *Pediatric Journal of Infectious Diseases.* 1993;12:664–71.

Goodwin M. "Managing nausea and vomiting of pregnancy." *Nutrition & the M.D.* Vol. 27,6, 2001.

Groziak SM, Kirksey A. "Effects of maternal dietary restriction in Vitamin B-6 on neocortex development of rats." *Journal of Nutrition.* 117: 1045–1052, 1987.

Guilarte TR. "Regional changes in the concentrations of glutamate, glycine, taurine, and GABA in the Vitamin B-6 deficient developing rat brain: association with neonatal seizures." *Neurochemistry Research.* 14: 889–97, 1989.

Harer WB. "Patient Choice Cesarean." *ACOG Clinical Review* 5(2):1, 13–16, 2000.

Haverkamp AD, Thompson HE, McFee JG, et al. "The evaluation of continuous fetal heart rate monitoring in high-risk pregnancy." *American Journal of Obstet. & Gynecol.* 125:310–20, 1976.

Haverkamp, AD, Orleans M, Langendoerfer S, et al. "A controlled trial of differential effects of intrapartum fetal monitoring." *American Journal of Ostet. & Gynecol.* 134:399–412, 1979.

Hourihan JO, Dean TP, Werner JO. "Peanut Allergy in relation to heredity, maternal diet, and other atopic diseases..." *British Medical Journal.* 313:518–21, 1996.

Hurtado KE, Claussen AH, Scott KG. "Early childhood anemia and mild or moderate mental retardation." *American Journal of Clinical Nutrition.* 69:115–119, 1999.

Kalliomaki M., et al. *The Lancet.* 357:1076–1079, 2001.

Kirksey A, Wachs TD, Yunis F, et al. Relation of maternal zinc nutriture to pregnancy outcome and infant Development in an Egyptian village." *American Journal of Clinical Nutrition.* 60:782–92, 1994.

Klaus MH, Kennel JH, Klaus PH. *Mothering the Mother: How a Doula Can Help You Have a Shorter, Easier, and Healthier Birth.* New York, Addison-Wesley. 1993.

Lede RL. "Is routine use of episiotomy justified?" *American Journal of Obstet. & Gynecol.* 69:687–95, 1987.

Levine EM, Ghai V, Barton JJ, et al. "Mode of Delivery and Risk of Respiratory Diseases in Newborns." *Obstet Cynecol.* 97:439–442, 2001.

Lu JY, Cook DL, Javia JB, et al. "Intakes of vitamins and minerals by pregnant women with selected Clinical symptoms." *Journal American Dietetic Association.* 78:477–82, 1981.

Lucas A, Morley R, Cole TJ et al. "Breast milk and subsequent intelligence quotient in children born Preterm." *Lancet.* 339:261–64, 1992.

Lucas A, Morley R, Cole TJ et al. "Early diet in preterm babies and developmental status at 18 months." *Lancet.* 335:1477–81, 1990.

McClure VS. *Infant Massage: A Handbook for Loving Parents.* New York: Bantam Doubleday Dell Pub. 2000.

McCullough AL, Kirksey A, Wachs TD, et al. "Vitamin B$_6$ status of Egyptian mothers: relation to infant behavior and maternal infant interactions." *American Journal of Clinical Nutrition.* 51:1067–74, 1990.

Newnham, JP. "Effects of frequent ultrasound during pregnancy: a randomized controlled study." *Lancet.* October 9, 1993: Vol. 342: 887–91.

Paul RH, Hon EH. "Clinical fetal monitoring: effect on perinatal outcome." *American Journal of Obstet. & Gynecol.* 188:529–33, 1974.

Rasmussen, K. Experimental Biology Meeting (Orlando: April 2001).

Reynolds, RD, Polansky M, Mosser PB. "Analyzed Vitamin B$_6$ intakes of pregnant and non-lactating women." *Journal American Dietetic Association.* 84:1339–44, 1984.

Reynolds, Robert D. "Perinatal Vitamin B$_6$ deficiency and poverty- is there are link?" *Nutrition Today.* Vol. 35, no. 6: 222–229, 2000.

Richardson AJ, et al. "Fatty acid metabolism in neuro-developmental disorders: a new perspective on associations between attention deficit disorders, dyslexia, dysperexia, and the autism spectrum." *Prostoglandins Leukot. Essential Fatty Acids.* 63(1/2): 1–9, 2000

Robson LC, Schwarz MR. "Vitamin B$_6$ deficiency and the lymphoid system. Effects of Vitamin B$_6$ deficiency in utero on the immunological competence of the offspring." *Cell Immunology.* 16:145–52, 1975.

Sampson HA, Mendelson L, Rosen JP. "Fatal or near-fatal anaphylactic reactions to food in children and adolescents." *New England Journal of Medicine.* 327:380–4, 1992.

Vadasp W Y, Burks W, Perelman B. "Detection of peanut allergens in breast milk of lactating women." *Journal of the American Medical Association.* 285:1746–8, 2001.

CHAPTER 11

Centers for Disease Control and Prevention website @ *http.//www.cdc.gov/nci-dod/eid.*

Centers for Disease Control. "Multistate surveillance for food handling, preparation, and consumption." *Morbidity & Mortality Weekly Report.* 47(55–4):33–57, 1998.

Centers for Disease Control. "Incidence of Foodborne Illness: preliminary data from the Foodborne Disease Active Surveillance Network (FoodNet)." *Morbidity & Mortality Weekly Report.* 48:189–94, 1999.

Duerr, K. *Doctor Mom's Quick Reference Guide to Natural Healthcare at Home.* Portland, OR: K. Duerr, 1998.

Duncan AL. *Your Healthy Child – A Guide to Natural Health Care.* Neskowin, OR: Sanicula Press, 1995.

Fan AM, Jackson RJ. "Pesticides and Food Safety." *Regulatory Toxicology & Pharmacology.* 9:158–74, 1989.

Guillette, E.A. et al. "An Anthropological approach to the evaluation of pre-school children exposed to pesticides in Mexico." *Environmental Health Perspectives.* June 106(6):347–53, 1998.

"How Safe is your Drinking Water?" *NOHA News.* Vol. XXVI, No. 3, Summer 2001, pp. 1–3.

Korich DG, Mead JR, Madore MS, et al. "Effects of ozone, chlorine dioxide, chlorine, and monochloramine on cryptosporidiumparvum oocyst viabil-ity." *Applied Environmental Microbiology.* 56:1423–8, 1990.

Lust J. *The Herb Book.* NY: Bantam Books/ published by arrangement with Benedict Lust Publications, 1974.

McGinn, AP. "Why poison ourselves? A precautionary approach to synthetic chemicals." *Worldwatch Paper.* 2000:153.

Millichap, J. Gordon. *Is our Water Safe to Drink? A Guide to Drinking Water Hazards and Health Risks.* Chicago: PNB Publishers, 1995.

Natural Resources Defense Council (NRDC). *Bottled Water: Pure Drink or Pure Hype?* 2000; website @ *www.nrdc.org/water/drinking/nbw.asp.*

Porter K, et al. "Pesticide health effects in drinking water." *Natural Resources Cornell Cooperative Extension.* 1998; website @ *www.pmep.cce.cornell.edu/facts-slides-self/facts/pes-heef-grw85.*

Potera, Carol. "Drugged drinking water." *Environmental Health Perspectives.* 2000; 108(10): A446.

"Twentieth Century Nutrition Review- Public Health Nutrition and Food Safety 1900-1999." *Nutrition Reviews.* Vol. 57, No. 12: 368–372.

U.S. Bureau of the Census. *Statistical Abstract of the United States,* 1995. Washington, D.C.: U.S. Bureau of the Census; 155th edition, 1995.

U.S. Environmental Protection Agency (EPA), Office of Ground Water and Drinking Water Programs. EPA Safe Drinking Water Hotline @ 1-800-426-4791; website at *www.epa.gov/safewater/mcl.htm.*

Zand J, Walton R, Roundtree, B. *Smart Medicine for a Healthier Child.* Garden City Park, NY: Avery Publishing Group. 1994.

CHAPTER 12

Blake, MS, RD, Joan Salge. "Healthy Snacks for Kids," *Thrive Online.com.* April, 1999.

Casa, DJ et al., National Athletic Trainers Association Position Statement: "Fluid replacement for athletes" *Journal of Athletic Training.* 2000; 35: 2/21.

Clark MS, RD, Nancy. *Nancy Clark's Sports Nutrition Guidebook.* 2nd ed. Massachusetts: Human Kinetics, 1997.

Coleman, R.D., M.A., M.P.H. and Steen, D.Sc., R.D., Suzzane Nelson. *The Ultimate Sports Nutrition Handbook*. California: Bull Publishing Company, 1996.

Convertino, VA et al., American College of Sports Medicine position stand: "Exercise and fluid replacement," *Medicine and Science in Sports and Exercise*. 1996; 28 il.

Di Pasquale M. *Nonessential of dispensible amino acids. In: Amino Acids and Proteins for the Athlete – The Anabolic Edge*. Boca Raton: CRC Press, 1997.

"Drink Up!" *The Nemours Foundation www.nemours.org* The Nemours Foundation Inc., 2000.

Duyff, M.S., R.D., C.F.C.S. *The American Dietetic Association's Complete Food & Nutrition Guide*. Minnesota: Chronimed Publishing, 1998.

"Eat Extra Calories For Excellence." *The Nemours Foundation www.nemours.org*. The Nemours Foundation Inc., 2000.

"Edible Energy." *The Nemours Foundation www.nemours.org*. The Nemours Foundation Inc., 2000.

Hass, M.D. Elson M. *Staying Healthy with Nutrition*. California: Celestial Arts, 1992.

Kelner, Jenny. "If Hectic Days Make Meals Impossible Try These Nutrition Packed Snacks," *Sports Parents Magazine*. 1995.

Leddy, M.D., John J., Pendergast, EdD, David R., and Venkatraman, PhD, Jaya T. "A Perspective of Fat Intake in Athletes," *Journal of American College of Nutrition* 19:3 (2000): 345–350.

Meduski JW. "The biochemistry and pharmacology of picolinic acid." Unpublished report, 1998.

Seal CJ. "Influence of dietary picolinic acid on mineral metabolism in the rat." *Am Nutr Metab*. 32: 186-91, 1988.

Takeuchi H et al. "Supplemental effects of arginine and methionine on growth, and on formations of urea and creatine of adrenalectomized rats fed high glycine diets." *Agr Biol Chem*. 39(5): 931–38, 1975.

CHAPTER 13

Astor, Stephen. *Hidden Food Allergies*. Garden City Park, NY: Avery Publishing Group, 1989.

Benton, D. "Dietary sugar, hyperactivity, and cognitive functioning: a methodological review." *J. Appl Nutr*. 41 (1):13–22. 1989.

Black, Dean. "Diet and Behavior." *The Healing Current Series*. Springville, UT: Tapestry Press, 1989.

Boris, M. & Mandel, F. "Foods and additives are common causes of the attention deficit hyperactive Disorder in children." *Annals of Allergy*. 72(5):462–7, 1993

Brin, M. "Behavioral effects of energy and protein deficits." DHEW (NIH) publication no. 79-1966, Washington D.C.: Department of Health, Education and Welfare, 1973.

Brocksmith, Carolyn Gallagher. "New diet can eliminate attention deficit disorder." *Opinion*. August 26, 1999.

Buist, Robert. *Food Chemical Sensitivity*. Garden City Park, NY: Avery Publishing Group, Inc., 1998.

Campbell, Bill. "Control Hyperactivity Naturally." *Better Nutrition*. pp. 14, 30, June 1989.

Condemi, John J. "Aspirin and Food Dye Reactions." *Bulletin of the New York Academy of Medicine*. Vol. 57, pp. 600-607, September 1981.

Conners, C.K. *Food Additives and Hyperactive Children*. New York: Plenum Press, pp. 107, 110; 1980.

Egger, Joseph. "The Hyperkinetic Syndrome." *Food Allergy and Intolerance, London: Medical Press.* pp. 674–686, 1987.

Egger, J. et al. "Controlled trial of oligoantigenic treatment in the hyperkinetic syndrome." *Lancet.* 1:540–5, 1985.

Egger, J., Carter, C.M. " A dietary management of severe child migraine." *Human Nutrition, Applied Nutrition.* 39A: 294–303, 1985.

Feingold, BF. "Hyperkinesis and learning disabilities linked to ingestion of artificial food colors and flavors." *J Learn Disabil.* 9(9):551–9, 1976.

Feingold, Ben F. *Why Your Child is Hyperactive.* New York: Random House, 1985.

Feingold, Helene, & Feingold, Ben. *The Feingold Cookbook for Hyperactive Children and Others with Problems Associated with Food Additives and Salicylates.* New York: Random House, 1979.

Firestone, P. et al. "The effects of caffeine on hyperactive children." *J Learn Disabil.* 11(3):133–141, 1978.

Fisher, Marjorie. "Foods and Chemicals Can Make Children Ill." *NOHA News.* Fall 1992. Vol. XVII, No. 4.

Galler, JR. "Malnutrition-a neglected cause of learning failure." *Postgrad Med.* 80:225–30, 1986.

Goldman, JA. Et al. "Behavioral effects of sucrose on preschool childen." *J Abnorm Child Psychol.* 14(4):65–77, 1986.

Gordon, S. "Junk food linked to low test scores." *The Modesto Bee* (California), November 16, 1986, p. 1.

Gross, M.D. "Effect of sucrose on hyperkinetic children." *Pediatrics.* 74(5): 76-7, 1984.

Haley, J.P., Ray, R.S., Tomasi, L. et al. "Hyperkinesis and food additives: testing the Feingold hypothesis." *Pediatrics.* 1978:61:818–28.

Hesser, Lynn. "Tartrazine on Trial." *Food and Chemical Toxicology.* Vol. 22, Dec 1984, pp. 1019–1024.

Hunter, Beatrice Trum. *Consumer Beware!* New York: Charles Scribner's and Sons, 1976.

Jacobson, MF. "Effects of sugar on behavior in children." Letter. *JAMA.* 275(10):756–7, 1996.

Kaplan, H.K. et al. "Behavioral effects of dietary sucrose in disturbed children." Letter to the editor. *Am J. Psychiat.* 143(7):944–945, 1986.

LeRiche, W. Harding. *A Chemical Feast.* New York: Facts on File Publications, 1982.

Lesser, M. *Nutrition and Vitamin Therapy.* New York: Bantam Books, 1980.

Lester ML et al. "Refined carbohydrate intake, hair cadmium levels and cognitive functioning in children." *Nutr Behav.* 1:3–13, 1982.

Lewis, Lisa. *Special Diets for Special Kids: Implementing a Diet to Improve the Lives of Children with Autism and Related Disorders.* Future Horizons, 1988.

Liebman, Bonnie. " The All-American Junk Food Diet." *Nutrition Action Newsletter.* May 1988, p. 8.

Magu, Joseph A., Tu, Anthony T. *Food Additive Toxicology.* New York: Marcel Dekker, Inc., 1995.

Mahan, K et al., "Sugar Allergy and Childrens' Behavior." *Abstract. Immunology and Allergy Practice,* July 1985, p. 81.

Maher, Timothy J. "Neurotoxicology of Food Additives." *Neurotoxicology.* v. 7, pp. 183–196, Summer 1986.

McGee, Charles. *How to Survive Modern Technology.* New cannan: Keats, 1979.

Messina, Virginia. "Is NutraSweet Safe?" *Pure Facts Newsletter of the Feingold Associations of the United States.* Vol. 14, No. 3, April 1990.

Milich, R., Wolraich, M, Lindgren, S. "Sugar and hyperactivity: a critical review of empirical findings." *Clin Psychol Rev.* 6:493–513, 1986.

Mindell, Earl. *Unsafe at Any Meal*. New York: Warner Books, 1987.

Moses, Susan. "Food Coloring May Alter Kids' Behavior." *The APA Monitor*. October 1989.

Mu-oz, KA, et al. "Food intakes of U.S. children and adolescents compared with recommendations." *Pediatrics*. 1997 Sep; 100(3):323–9.

Nelson, M. "Workshop on 'nutrition and the school child' – food, vitamins and IQ" *Proc Nutr Soc*. 50:29-35, 1991.

Olney, John W. "Excitatory neurotoxins as Food Additives: An Evaluation of Risk." *Neurotoxicology*. v. 2, pp. 163–192, January 1981.

Perara, Judith. "Authorities Ban Food Coloring from School Dinners." *New Scientist*. v. 111, 8/14/86, p. 14.

Prinz, R.J. et al. "Dietary correlates of hyperactive behavior in children." *J. Consulting Clin. Psychol*. 48:760–9, 1980.

Pure Facts. Newsletter of the Feingold Associations of the United States. (ongoing newsletter with specific references to salicytate-free diets of autism, ADD, ADHD, and Learning disabilities.)

Rapp, Doris J. *Allergies and the Hyperactive Child*. New York: Sovereign Books, 1979.

Rowe, Katherine & Rowe, Kenneth. "Synthetic food coloring and behavior, a dose response effect in a double-blind, placebo-controlled, repeated measures study." *J Pediatrics*. 125:691: 8, 1994.

Sadler, M.J. "Recent Aspartame Studies." *Food and Chemical Toxicology*. v. 22, 9/84, pp. 771–773.

Salamy, J. et al. "Physiological Changes in Hyperactive Children Following the Ingestion of Food Additives." *International Journal of Neuroscience*. Vol 16, pp. 241-246, May 1982.

Schecter, MD, Gibbons, GD. "Objectively measured hyperactivity. II. Caffeine and amphetamine effects." *J Clin Pharmacol*. 1985.25:276–80.

Schmidt, M.A. *Smart Fats: How Dietary Fats and Oils Affect Mental, Physical and Emotional Intelligence*. Frog, Ltd., 1997.

Schmidt, M.H. et al. "Does oligoantigenic diet influence hyperactive/ conduct-disordered children – a controlled trial." *Eur Child Adolesc Psychiatry*. 6(2):88–95, 1997.

Schoeder, HA. "Losses of vitamins and trace minerals resulting from processing and preservation of foods." *Am J Clin Nutr*. 24:562–73, 1971.

Schoenthaler, Stephen J. "Sugar and children's behavior." *The New England Journal of Medicine*. Vol. 330, No. 26, pp. 1901–4, June 30, 1994.

Schoenthaler, Stephen J., Walter E. Doraz, and James A. Wakefield, Jr. "The Impact of a Low Food Additive and Sucrose Diet on Academic Performance in 803 New York City Public Schools." *Int. J. Biosocial Research*. 8(2):185–195, 1986.

Schoenthaler, Stephen J., Walter E. Doraz, and James A. Wakefield, Jr. "The Testing of Various Hypotheses as Explanations for the Gains in National Standardized Academic Test Scores in the 1978–1983 New York City Nutrition Policy Modification Project." *Int. J Biosocial Research*. Vol. 8(2): 196–203, 1986.

South, J. "Natural Remedies for ADD." *Nutritional News*. 11(9), September 1997.

Spring, B. & Wurtman, RJ. "Effects of food and nutrients on the behavior of normal individuals." In: Wurtman JJ, editor. *Nutrition and the Brain*. Volume 7. New York: Raven Press; 1985. p. 1–47.

Stevens, L, et al. "Essential fatty acids in boys with attention-deficit hyperactivity disorder." *Am J Clin Nutr*. 62:761–8, 1995.

"Study links sugar, child anxiety." *Chicago Tribune*. May 10, 1990.

Swain, A. et al. "Salicylates, oligoantigenic diets, and behavior." Letter to the editor. *Lancet*. pp. 41–42, July 6, 1985.

Swanson, J.M. and M. Kinsbourne. "Artificial food colors impair the learning of hyperactive children." *Report to the Nutrition Foundation*. 482 Fifth Avenue, New York, NY, 1979.

"Sweet Talk." *Scientific American*. Vol 257, p. 16, July 1987.

TePas, Theodore E. "Hyperactivity Revisited." *Noha News*. Winter 1988, Vol. XIII, No. 1.

Turnlund, JR et al. "Vitamin B_6 depletion followed by repletion with animal- or plant-source diets and calcium and magnesium metabolism in y oung women." *Am J Clin Nutr*. 56:905–910. 1992.

Weiss, Bernard. "Food additives as a source of behavioral disturbances in children." *Neurotoxicology*. Vol. 7, pp. 197–208, Summer 1986.

Wender, E. "Review of research on the relationship of nutritive sweeteners and behavior." In: *Diet and Behavior*. Washington, D.C.: National Center for Nutrition and Dietetics, 65-80, 1991.

White, JW. And M. Wolraich. "Effect of sugar on behavior and mental performance." *Am J Clin Nutr*. 62(suppl):242S–98, 1995.

Winter, Ruth. *A Consumer's Dictionary of Food Additives*. New York: Crown, 1984.

Wolraich, M.L. et al. "Effects of diets high in sucrose or aspartame on the behavior and cognitive performance of children." *The New England Journal of Medicine*. Vol. 330, No. 5, pp. 301-307.

Wolraich, M. et al. "Effects of sucrose ingestion on the behavior of hyperactive boys." *J. Pediatrics*. 106(4):675–82, 1985.

Wolraich, ML et al. "The effect of sugar on behavior or cognition in children." *JAMA*. 274:1617–21, 1995.

Wood, David et al. "The Prevalence of Attention Deficit Disorder, Residual Type, or Minimal Brain Dysfunction, In a Population of Male Alcoholic Patients." *Am. J. Psychiatry*. 140(1):95–98, 1983.

Woodbury, MM, Woodbury, MA. "Neuropsychiatric development: two case reports about the use of dietary fish oils and/or chronic dietary supplements in children. *J Am Coll Nutr*. 12(3):239–45, 1993.

Wurtman, RJ. "Neurochemical changes following high-dose aspartame with dietary carbohydrates." *N. Engl J Med*. 309:429–30, 1983.

Yokogoski, Hidehoke et al. "Effects of Aspartame and Glucose Administration on Brain Plasma Levels of Large Neutral Amino Acids and brain 5-Hydroxindoles." *American Journal of Clinical Nutrition*. v. 40, July '84, pp. 1–7.

Zametkin, A.J., and J.L. Rappaport. "Neurobiology of Attention Deficit Disorder with Hyperactivity: Where Have We Come in 50 Years?" *J. Acad.Child and Adol. Psychiat*. 26:676–86, 1987.

Zimmerman, Marcia. "Facing Attention Deficit Disorders." *Nutrition Science News*. Vol.3., No. 10, October 1998

CHAPTER 14

Alaimo K, McDowell MA, et al. "Dietary intake of vitamins, minerals, and fiber of persons ages 2 months and over in the U.S.," No. 258. Hyattsville, MD: *National Center of Health Statistics*. 1994.

Albertson AM, Tobelman RC, Engstrom A, et al. "Nutrient intakes of 2–10 year old American children: 10 year trends." *Journal of the American Dietetic Association*. 92:1492-6, 1992

American Academy of Pediatrics; website @ *www.aap.org*. and 2000 Annual Meeting.

Birch LL, Marlin DW, Rotter J. " Eating as the "means" activity in a contingency: Effects on young children's food preference." *Child Development.* 55:423–439, 1984.

Birch LL, Johnston SL, Fisher JA. "Children's eating: the development of food acceptance patterns." *Young Children.* 50:71–78, 1995.

Birch LL, Marlin DW. "I don't like it; I never tried it: Effects of exposure on two-year old children's food preferences." *Appetite.* 3:353–360, 1982.

Black R, Sazawal S, Shankar A. "Reduction of Pneumonia and Diarrhea worldwide with zinc supplements." *Journal of Pediatrics.* December 2000.

Carruth BR, Skinner J, et al. "The Phenomenon of 'picky eater:' A behavioral marker in eating patterns of toddlers." *Journal of the American College of Nutrition.* Vol. 17, No. 2: 180–186, 1998.

Centers for Disease Control, "Breast-fed babies need Vitamin D", website @ *www. cdc.gov/ncidod/eid.* 2001.

Contento I, Balch GI, et al. "The effectiveness of nutrition education and implications for nutrition education policy, programs, and research." *Journal of Nutritional Education.* 27:279–83, 1995.

Cox DR, Skinner J, Carruth BR, et al. "A variety index for toddlers (VTT: Development and application)." *Journal of the American Dietetic Association.* 97: 1382–1386, 1997.

Crane NT, Hubbard VS, Lewis CT. "American diets and year 2000 goals." *U.S. Department of Agriculture Information Bulletin.* No. 750, 1999.

Crayhon, Robert. *Nutrition Made Simple: A Comprehensive Guide to the Latest Findings in Optimal Nutrition.* New York: M. Evans and Co., 1996.

Eden AN, Mir M. "Iron deficiency in 1–3 year old children – a pediatric failure?" *Arch Pediatric Adolesc Med.* 151:986, 1997.

Eden A. "Iron Deficiency and the Toddler: An Ongoing Dilemna." *Nutrition & the M.D.* Vol. 27, No. 1, pp. 1–3, January 2001.

Florencio, C. "Developments and Variations in School-Based feeding programs around the world." *Nutrition Today.* Vol. 36, No. 1: 29–42.

"Fortified Toddlers," *TIME.* January 31, 2000, p. 84.

Halterman, J. "Mild Iron deficiency linked with low math scores." *Journal of Pediatrics.* June 2001.

Hurtado EK, Claussen AH, Scott KG. "Early childhood anemia and mild or moderate mental retardation." *American Journal Clinical Nutrition.* 69:115–119, 1999.

Kant, A. et al. "Junk food eating habits causing long-term health consequences," *JAMA.* 283:2109–2115, 2000.

Karjalainen S. et al. "Toddler's snacks predict cavities at age six," *Dentistry and Oral Epidemiology.* 29:136–142, 2001.

Kinter M, Boss P, Johnson N. "The relationship between dysfunctional family environments and family member food intake." *Journal of Marriage and Family.* 43:633–641, 1983.

Lloyd T, Andon MB et al. "Calcium supplementation and bone mineral density in adolescent girls." *JAMA.* 1993:270:841–8446.

Looker AC, Dallman PR, Carroll MD, et al. "Prevalence of iron deficiency in the U.S." *JAMA.* 13:521–37, 1997.

Lozoff B, Jimenez E, Wolf AW. "Long-term developmental outcomes of infants with iron deficiency." *New England Journal of Medicine.* 325: 687–94.

Lozoff B, et al. "Iron deficiency anemia and iron therapy: Effects on infant developmental test performance." *Pediatrics.* 79:981, 1987.

McBean L, Miller GD. "Enhancing the Nutrition of America's Youth." *Journal of the American College of Nutrition.* Vol. 18, No. 6: 563–571, 1999.

Pelchat ML, Pliner D. "Antecedents and Correlates of feeding problems in young children." *Journal of Nutritional Education.* 18:23–29, 1986.

Picciano MF et al. "Nutritional guidance is needed during dietary transition in early childhood." *Pediatrics.* 106:109, 2000.

Pliner P, Pelchat M, Grapski M. "Reduction of neophobia in humans by exposure to novel foods." *Appetite.* 20:111–123. 1993.

Pollitt E. "Iron deficiency and cognitive function." *Annual Review of Nutrition.* 13:521–37, 1993.

Prentice A. "Calcium requirements of children." *Nutritional Review.* 53: 37–45, 1995.

"Probiotics reduce diarrhea in hospitalized children." *Journal of Pediatrics.* 138:361–5, 2001.

Roberts S, Heyman M, Mayer J. "Micronutrient shortfalls in young children's diets: Common and owing inadequate intakes both at home and at child care centers." *Nutrition Reviews.* Vol. 58, No. 1, pp. 27–29, 2000.

Simopolous, A. "Genetic Variation and Nutrition." *Nutrition Reviews.* Vol 5, No. 5, S10–S19, May 1999.

Skinner J, Carruth BR, Houck K, et al. "Transitions in infant feeding in the first year of life." *Journal of the American College of Nutrition.* 16: 209–215, 1997.

Sullivan SA, Birch LL. "Infant dietary experience and acceptance of solid foods." *Pediatrics.* 93:271–278, 1993.

U.S. Department of Health & Human Services, Public Health Service: Healthy People 2000, Hyattsville MD: National Center for Health Statistics, 1995.

Walravens PA, Hambidge KM. "Growth of infants fed a zinc supplement formula." *Am J Clin Nutr.* 29:1114–21, 1976.

Walravens PA, Krebs NF, Hambidge KM. "Linear growth of low income preschool children receiving a zinc supplement." *Am J Clin Nutr.* 38: 195–201, 1983.

Walter T et al. "Effects of mild iron deficiency on infant mental development scores." *Journal of Pediatrics.* 102:519, 1983.

Yates AA, Schlicker SA, Suitor CW. "Dietary reference intakes: the new brains for recommendations for calcium and related nutrients, B vitamins, and cholene." *Journal of American Dietetic Association.* 92:1492–6, 1992.

CHAPTER 15

Borba, Michelle. *Parents Do Make a Difference: How to Raise Healthy Kids with Solid Character, Strong Minds, and Caring Hearts.* New York: Jossey Bass, 2000.

Brazelton, T. Berry, M.D. *Touchpoints: The Essential Reference.* New York: Addison-Wesley Publishing Company, 1992.

Gibbs, Nancy. "Who's in charge there? Do kids have too much power? *TIME.* pp. 40–49, August 6, 2001.

Hart, Betsy. "Kids need parents who know how to say no." *Chicago Sun-Times.* August 15, 2001.

Kindlon, Dan. *Too Much of a Good Thing: Raising Children of Character in an Indulgent Age.* Talk Miramax.

Williams, Reid. "Parents pave way to smarter kids." *Pioneer Press – Back to School.* August 2, 2001, p. 1.

CONCLUSION REFERENCES

"Junk Diets: Damage Report." *Nutrition Action Health Letter.* p. 13, Jan/Feb 2001.

"Junk Food undermining school meal plans." *The Nation's Health.* April 2001.

Kant, Ashima et al. *JAMA.* 283:2109-2115, 2000.

Kant, Ashima et al. "One-third of the American diet is junk food." *American Journal of Clinical Nutrition.* 72:929–936, 2000.

"Public health bills may be winners in senate upset." *The Nation's Health.* July 2001.

INDEX

269

OUR CHILDREN'S HEALTH

America is in the throes of a nutritional crisis – and children are at its very heart.

Here is a book that forthrightly examines this problem from the perspective of an internationally renowned nutritionist and a holistically trained physician.

Learn why:

- 1 out of every 5 American children is overweight.
- The incidence of asthma has increased 61% in the past 20 years.
- Increased teen violence may be attributable to the prescribed use of some antidepressant drugs.
- Immunizations may be related to autism in infants and children.
- 2 out of 5 of today's teenagers are likely to later develop osteoporosis.
- Environmental and food toxins may cause neurological and behavioral problems.
- Commonly prescribed amphetamines are <u>not</u> the answer to ADHD.
- Eating disorders amond near epidemic proportions.

The authors present a positive, balanced approach to health and nutrition that addresses these issues and offers hope to millions of undernourished, overmedicated children and their families.

There are few topics that are as important to the long-term well-being of our culture as the health of our children.... Bonnie Minsky and Lisa Holk provide a thorough current review of some of the major issues contributing to this problem along with many practical action items you can take to make sure your children can achieve their maximum health.

JOSEPH MERCOLA, D.O., FOUNDER AND DIRECTOR OF WWW.MERCOLA.COM

Bonnie Minsky and Dr. Lisa Holk have written a book that is eminently readable and well researched, and that addresses the issue of what to feed our children in a direct and straight-forward manner. They have accepted the challenge of making this wealth of information available in a practical way, so that parents can learn to understand why their children are not well, and how to rectify the situation.

RITA BETTENBURG, N.D.

This book abounds with choices of natural medicine and treatments for children. It is a remarkable contribution that will enlighten and empower parents and practitioners alike.

TONY V. LU, M.D., MEDICAL DIRECTOR,
INTEGRATIVE MEDICINE, LOYOLA UNIVERSITY HEALTH SYSTEM

VITAL HEALTH PUBLISHING

Health ~ Nutrition

$15.95

ISBN: 1-890612-27-8